To Elizabeth Tasse –
　　　With affection and admiration!

　　　　　Carla Chen

April 1997

*Demand and Get
the Best
Health Care
for You*

Demand and Get the Best Health Care for You

An Eminent Doctor's Practical Advice

Curtis Prout, M.D.

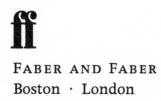

FABER AND FABER
Boston · London

First published in the United States in 1996 by
Faber and Faber, Inc., 53 Shore Road, Winchester, MA 01890

Prout, Curtis, 1915–
    Demand and get the best health care for you: an eminent
doctor's practical advice / Curtis Prout.
        p.   cm.
    ISBN 0-571-19896-1 (cloth)
    1. Medical care.   2. Consumer education.   I. Title.
RA410.5.P76   1996
362.1 — dc20   96-15743
                                                        CIP

To everyone,
who sooner or later will suffer in some way,
and to those who wish to help.

Contents

Foreword

America's health-care system is a huge and complex enterprise. It is changing rapidly under the impact of unprecedented economic forces and a great variety of new social, cultural, and political trends. Always a mystery to most laypersons, and even to many health professionals working in it, our health-care system has now become even more difficult to understand. How is health care funded and insured? In what institutional organizations and by what kinds of professional personnel is heath care delivered? Most of us will sooner or later put our own health—and quite possibly our lives—in the hands of this system, so what should we know about it that will increase our chances of being effectively served?

These are some of the questions this practical, down-to-earth volume is designed to answer. Written by a senior and very wise clinician and medical teacher, it describes in simple and straightforward terms the essential elements of our health-care system and how they work. It also gives helpful advice on how to make the best use of the system—how to choose the right physicians or other health-care providers, and the right health-care institutions.

Dr. Prout has written a primer for patients that will be of interest to anyone seeking a brief, clear introduction to the present U.S.

health-care system. It deserves a wide readership and I hope that is what it gets. I doubt that all of his medical colleagues will agree with every one of his opinions in this book, but I am sure most will recognize that he has made a very valuable contribution.

ARNOLD S. RELMAN, M.D.
Editor-in-Chief Emeritus,
New England Journal of Medicine

Acknowledgments

So many people, so many conferences, so many journal and news-paper articles have contributed to the facts and opinions expressed in this book that no particular one can be singled out. In an infor-mal manner I tried to add up the number of teachers who have made a profound and lasting impression on me, and whose influ-ence I treasure, but I stopped counting after the first hundred. In-formal exchanges at meals, on vacation, and in the hospital corri-dors make, as Francis Bacon said, "a ready man," ready to follow up this important if subliminal education.

Patients, of all kinds and under an exceptional variety of circum-stances, have contributed even more. Their feelings and opinions form the matrix of this book into which are woven the enduring as well as the revolutionary new facts and ideas. Throughout, it can hardly be emphasized enough, is the relation between the patient and the doc-tor or nurse. We cannot listen enough to what patients feel and say.

Valerie Cimino, my editor, and her colleagues at Faber and Faber are patient, helpful, and admirably perfectionistic without exces-sively bruising the ego of the author.

Beth Nilsson, my tactful, skillful, and hard-working assistant, has cheerfully typed, retyped, and cajoled a mass of details into what I hope is a coherent whole.

Introduction

"How do I go about picking a doctor or a health plan?" a friend asked me recently. I had no quick, easy, or simple answer. There are lots of other questions as well.

What is the best health plan currently available? What is not covered by your health insurance? What reliable alternatives exist to the prevailing establishment system of care? Will you be able to learn about and receive the benefits of the latest research? What is managed care, and how does it affect these choices? Can I still have my own family doctor? The more you know of the process, the more complicated it seems.

The solutions are not going to be the same for each person. The search involves knowing what options are available to you and knowing as much as you can about each of them. Above all, this search must involve knowing yourself—what you need, what health-care needs you expect you will have, and how much or how little you need to rely on your doctor. These are some of the factors you must decide for yourself. This book is about helping you find your way.

Everyone wants a doctor whom they like, who can be easily reached by phone or in person, whom they can afford, who is covered by their insurance plan, who has a reputation for professional excellence, and who will take time to listen. This is a tall order, and it is not certain that many people will ever connect with such a paragon of virtues. Most of us hope, furthermore, that these goals can be achieved for everybody, without radically disturbing the American economy.

What is the justification for another book on health care and doctors today? The answer is that patients (or, in the current jargon, "health-care consumers") are almost without exception confused, anxious, and in many cases angry. Above all, people are looking for information, not the rhetoric seen in health-plan advertisements, public-relations releases, or political speeches. The public's many concerns are emotional responses to a complex set of frustrations, each of which exists because of certain circumstances, customs, and social and economic forces. It can be frightening not to have a system on which you can count to take care of your concerns in a reliable, affordable, and caring way. Perhaps "system" is not an appropriate word to describe American health care; "nonsystem" or even "rampant pluralism" would be a more fitting description. Doctors as well as patients are slowly accepting the new realities, one of which is that everyone will have to accept less than the ideal. Being honest and having a realistic outlook cannot fail to improve the situation. There is enough finger-pointing, name-calling, and over-simplified arguments. They will get us nowhere. People need to be alert, informed, and vigilant.

The average American likes his or her doctor. Patients worry, however, about the system, about losing their doctors, and about losing the choice of doctor or hospital. At present, increasing numbers of people have no established family doctor, whether primary-care family practitioner or general internist, and they are at a loss as to how to find the right one.

People seek medical care for few, but powerful, reasons: fear, pain, or anxiety. These may take many forms and have many causes, both physical and emotional. As Dr. Eric Cassell of Cornell Medical School has pointed out, the relief of suffering is the doctor's most important job. Unfortunately, the present trends in medical care—fragmentation of responsibility, restricted choices of caregivers and hospitals, and exorbitant costs—often increase rather than relieve this suffering. No one plan will work for everyone, because illness and health mean different things to different people. For example, to some, a sudden internal pain conjures up the fear of death, but to others these ominous possiblities are denied, and anything or any person bringing relief of symptoms is good enough. Geography, culture, family history, belief systems, and expectations make each person's attitude toward illness unique. The obvious first step, therefore, is to learn as much as you can about these factors as they relate to you.

Taking responsibility for your own health care is tedious and hard work, because in order to make an informed decision you need to study and understand the various medical systems and their financial structure; the ways doctors, nurses, clinics, and hospitals function; and the kinds of care available. Above all, you, the patient—the customer—should know what you really need, want, can afford, and can realistically expect. The more you know about yourself and how your body gets well and stays well, the less you will need to feel so dependent on a complicated system that is becoming larger and more fragmented all the time.

To help you make your health-care choices, I will try to put you, the reader, in the various shoes of the patient, the doctor, the nurse, and the administrator, in an effort to help you understand how and why things work.

You must take charge of your own health care if humanly possible, because only you can decide for yourself the relative importance of such things as accessibility, cost, quality of life, confidentiality, warm reassurance, and prolonging life.

1

What's Going On?

*It is difficult, indeed, for a layman in the city to find the
right physician if he has been so unfortunate as to have had
good health until some emergency arises.*

ROBERT T. MORRIS

To illustrate the enormity of people's concerns about health care,
here are just some of the things we hear every day.

Let's start with patients. Here is a list of various concerns and
gripes.

*"I like my doctor, but I hate the system" (or the American Medical Asso-
ciation, or the Social Security Administration, or the Veterans Administra-
tion, or Blue Cross, or US Healthcare).*
"How can I find a doctor I like and trust?"
"How can I find out the doctor's credentials?"
"Should I pick a doctor by his or her hospital affiliation?"
"Can I join a plan that gives me a choice of doctor?"
"I am paying more and getting less." (A laborer)

"I can't get to talk with my doctor, and if I do, he does not listen long enough." (A schoolteacher)

"If I want to see a specialist, why do I have to plead with my primary-care doctor or group?" (A professional woman)

"My anxieties and depression make my life not worth living, and I am unable to work, sleep, or get help."

"Anyway, doctors are rich and stick with their own social group. How can they understand my problems?" (An angry minority husband and father)

"I spend most of my time micromanaging my doctors." (A young woman with a rare type of arthritis)

"I don't like to be treated as if I don't know anything." (A minority woman)

"Why is my time worthless? Can't the doctor or clinic make appointments and stick to the schedule within reason?" (A person who loses pay by taking time off from work while waiting to be seen)

"Does the doctor know how much these medicines cost?" (A patient on high doses of a new antibiotic)

"I am taking medicines called Zantac, Zyloprim, Xanax, and Prozac. What on earth are they? How do I tell them apart?" (A patient with medicines for ulcer, gout, insomnia, and depression)

"I take a list of questions to the doctor to save him time and to be thorough, but the list seems to make him angry." (A lawyer)

"If I dye my hair, pierce my eyelids, or have a tattoo, should that tell the doctor that I am worthless and need a moral lecture?" (A high-school student)

"If I question the nurse practitioner about what seems to be an obvious mistake, I get severely reprimanded." (A conscientious, worried mother)

"The doctor's office is messy and crowded." (A young mother)

"I like to be addressed in the doctor's office as Mrs., not as Jane." (A grandmother)

"My doctor is too close and friendly, even nosy." (A clergyman)

"My doctor is too remote and impersonal." (Another clergyman)

"I am going to try alternative medicines. I hear they have some wonderful, new secret drug." (A cancer patient)

"Orthopedic specialists have not helped my back. Which is better, chiropractic, massage therapy, acupuncture, or Chinese medicine?" (A sufferer from chronic back pain)

"Can my coverage be changed or cancelled without my knowing? What preexisting conditions are not covered? My coverage has changed. How can I be sure what is still covered?" (A secretary in a law firm)

These are all actual statements, and in one version or another they are really universal concerns, yet many surveys have shown that most people are satisfied with their present medical care. Their satisfaction is not without reservations, however. For any illness or operation that has a good outcome, the relief and gratitude do not always make up for some unpleasant experiences along the way. This satisfaction is one of the many reasons that the Clinton health-care initiative failed to receive enough support.

Now, having heard what the patients say, let's listen to some of the concerns of doctors today.

"I can no longer have a career that permits professional growth and deep personal satisfaction without being overwhelmed by rules, paperwork, and continuous oversight." (An internist who is quitting practice to go to work for an insurance company)

"Why don't people know how hard I work and under what pressures?" (A private primary-care physician)

"I used to be respected and trusted. Now I feel on the defensive, and my work is criticized and second-guessed." (A prominent internist)

"Besides, I am earning a lot less than I used to." (Another generalist)

"After all my extra training and certification, why can't I get more work, and why has Medicare cut my fees by almost half?" (A board-certified cardiologist associated with a major teaching hospital)

"I'd like to order fewer tests, but my malpractice advisor suggests that I do even more." (An urban gastroenterologist)

"Since managed-care plans cannot prove that psychotherapy is cost-effective for their purposes, my patients have to pay all or most of the cost of their mental-health care." (A psychiatrist)

"I know that in my annual review at the health maintenance organization (HMO) where I work that I will be financially penalized for not seeing more patients in less time." (A conscientious generalist in a large managed-care practice)

One might expect that with concerns such as these, applications to medical schools would decrease. On the contrary, in the last three years there has been a dramatic increase in the number, and quality, of applicants to U.S. medical schools.

The nurses also have their complaints, and here are a few:

"I can't get a good job because I went to a 'diploma school' and don't have a bachelor's degree." (Private nurse doing home care)

"After earning a B.A. and an M.A. in nursing and keeping up my continuing-education credits, I still have to work under the orders of doctors, some of whom I do not think competent or up-to-date." (A thirty-five-year-old ward nurse in a large hospital)

"With all my special training and advanced education, I am now being replaced by a less-trained, lower-paid worker." (A hospital nurse)

"Some people still expect us, after all this training and supervision, to arrange flowers and empty bedpans." (A female nurse)

"Some people think we are failed doctors, inadequate persons, or even untrained orderlies." (A male R.N. in a hospital)

Hospitals, too, have their own problems and complaints. Many small cash-strapped hospitals can no longer meet mandated standards and have gone out of existence. Many communities want to keep their local hospitals open but cannot afford to do so. Rapid transportation and telecommunications are of considerable help in getting medical assistance and consultation to rural areas, thus making small local hospitals less essential. Larger hospitals, facing tighter restrictions on admissions and length of stay, have many empty beds. Their fixed expenses can be cut only partially by drastic reductions in staff and services. Many hospitals are merging with others to consolidate purchasing and eliminate competing services. One result of the newly expanding phenomenon of hospitals advertising their particular expertise to the public is that in the rush to get a larger share of the patient business, they compete not only with each other but even with physicians practicing in the community. Other hospitals are trying to operate convalescent homes, partly as a source of profit and partly to ensure a steady supply of ill, elderly patients. Others are buying out general and family practices to be sure these doctors send their patients to their hospital.

In short, money governs what hospitals can and cannot do. A committee of the trustees of a highly respected teaching hospital in Boston is at present considering whether under today's circumstances the hospital still deserves to be considered a tax-exempt charity. Since for-profit hospitals must pay taxes, the pressure to reexamine tax exemptions for all hospitals is growing.

Given all these concerns, we should listen to the people who are in actual fact determining the scope and direction of American medical care. For convenience's sake, let's call them as a group the money people. The executives, administrators, and investors in the rapidly growing for-profit managed-care systems have joined with the nonprofits, the "Blues," with hospital administrators, and with insurance companies to take control of health-care income and expenditures. The fact is that privatization of medical care and all of its branches has moved rapidly ahead, and as an industry, health care has been one of the most successful investments in recent years.

There have also been huge investments in the development of effective new drugs and huge profits in the pharmaceutical industry.

The History of Health Care

To understand how the changes in the health-care industry came about, almost without most people realizing it, consider history. From the beginning of this country to the period around World War II, physicians defined the terms and set the rules of health care, acting through their local and national medical societies and based on their teachings in medical schools. Physicians did the research, largely with private funding. Physicians set their own high research and educational standards. Starting in the 1940s, the hospitals, particularly the large urban teaching hospitals, the medical schools, and specialty societies, took over the power from physicians.

In 1940 approximately 95 percent of all American physicians were general practitioners. At present, only 40 percent of all new medical-school graduates go into general care. In the past fifty years, the specialists have written the rules, set the standards, and determined the medical-school curricula. Published research has been up to now the key to academic and financial promotion.

Passage of the Medicare and Medicaid Acts in 1965 and 1966, and the generous funding of hospital construction by the federal government in the Hill-Burton Act of 1946, among other changes, assured hospitals and medical schools of almost limitless expansion, with only modest fiscal restraint. In less than two years after the implementation of Medicare and Medicaid, the income of U.S. physicians doubled. The principal reason for this startling jump was political. The Congress, in order to persuade organized medicine that the doctors themselves would profit by accepting the changes involved in making care available to the elderly and the poor, assured these physicians that they would continue to receive their "usual and customary" fees. Many doctors promptly decided

that the previous charges were below the market, and indeed that a
$10 fee, for example, may have been usual but $20 was the true
"customary" value. More physicians joined the crowd, and soon
this rising tide lifted all the boats.

In addition to substantial federal contributions through various
agencies, principally the National Institutes of Health, states, cities,
private foundations, and wealthy individuals poured money into
research. Generous support for medical-school and hospital-based
research, with generous allowances for "overhead," made research
an attractive field for doctors. This brought prestige as well as
higher income to academic and specialized doctors and hospitals.
Until very recently, academic medicine was the tail that wagged the
dog of American health care, and the professors were the ruling
powers. There was a very good side to all of these changes. The constant advances in training and technology and the results of research, with the resulting rewards for excellence, made American
medicine and hospitals the envy of the world. For most physicians
who were active from 1950 to the 1980s this was, indeed, a golden
age, even if some minority and female physicians did not share the
full largesse and respect.

Eventually, the costs of paying for Medicare and Medicaid
teaching and research as well as advanced diagnostic equipment
caught up with the health-care industry.

Changes and Challenges

The reality of economic and social changes has brought about a
rapid and dramatic shift in power; most people have not been aware
of this over the past ten years. Health-care costs got out of hand.

1960	1993
$27 billion	$884 billion
67 percent paid privately	32 percent paid privately

The people and organizations who have underwritten the costs of health care deserve and demand control over it. An old proverb comes to mind: "He who pays the piper, calls the tune." Local, state, and federal funding agencies have joined with the private nonprofit agencies such as Blue Cross and Blue Shield, and the for-profit insurers, such as Travelers and Aetna, and giant health-care corporations such as Columbia and US Healthcare to take control. Physicians, nurses, hospitals, and medical schools must now follow the new rules or be put out of business, as some already have been.

Neither run-of-the-mill people (patients) nor actual run-of-the-mill practicing doctors were among the select and secret three hundred advisors on Clinton's proposed health-care plan. Further, despite their crocodile tears for the concerns of the common people and their troubles, the insurers, the for-profit health-care corporations, pharmaceutical manufacturers, and medical suppliers had their own agenda and spent millions of dollars in lobbying for their own interests. Since private investment is increasingly involved, it is obvious that executives are responsible to their stockholders, and their job is to maximize profit. Serving the consumer is of secondary interest at best. This is the American Way. As Calvin Coolidge once said, "The business of America is business."

What the patient will receive and what the patient will pay for health care in the future will be determined by the money people. But the future is too important to leave in the hands of the money people. Only a powerful voice, a sort of coalition, can help patients and their caregivers achieve what will certainly be a compromise. We cannot have everything. The kindly, friendly, all-knowing, ever-available, never tired, never harassed, poverty-stricken-but-proud Dr. Wonderful will never be seen again. As a matter of fact, he never did exist in real life. At the same time it is not realistic to expect congressmen, who have reelection always in mind, to bite the bullet and cut entitlements, limit options, or raise taxes, and it is not clear at this time how these obvious economies are going to be achieved. The public must do the best it can with what is currently in place, and always with a sharp eye on legislative changes, and write their representatives when necessary.

We live in angry times, but anger is no way to solve our health-care problems. The worst outcome is to have patients and caregivers angry at and blaming each other. Not only is this destructive; worse yet, it diverts our efforts away from our common goal, which is an acceptable level of competent care for everyone at a cost that workers and other taxpayers can bear. It is helpful to remember that patients will always need doctors and vice versa. If everyone makes an effort to understand why things are the way they are, there is hope that patients and doctors can together help establish a system that will satisfy the greatest number of people.

To understand what is going on with health care, it is necessary to reemphasize that patients and doctors no longer are in control of the health-care system, and that this turn of events reflects larger systemic developments. To quote the editor of the *New England Journal of Medicine*, Dr. Jerome Kassirer, "I suspect that the embracing of market values in health care reflects a change in society as a whole. Because individualism and competition are increasingly celebrated, the principles of the market place now permeate our personal lives and even capture our judgment. When we spend our waking hours scheming about how to win, it becomes difficult to keep in touch with fundamental human needs." He goes on to point out that there have been some good results coming from managed care, for instance, the curbing of excessive testing and unnecessary treatment and the shortening of hospital stays, and other methods of eliminating "redundant layers of bureaucracy and wasteful paperwork." He further states that "leaders should also acknowledge that managing care can limit costs. But they should go on to say that the enormous profits of megahospital systems and huge insurance conglomerates should be used for medical care. Until they are we have not tried hard enough to discover whether our resources are sufficient to reverse restrictions in care. A rich country like ours that spends nearly a trillion dollars a year on health care and enormous sums on tobacco, alcohol, and cosmetics should be able to meet the basic health needs of its citizens."

Downsizing and consolidation of hospitals will undoubtedly continue at a frantic pace as a way for institutions to save money. The unanswered question is whose money is saved? It is time to take a hard look at the hidden costs of day surgery, of early hospital discharge after illness or delivery, and of reducing the ratio of nurses to patients. Already several states have passed legislation directing insurers to pay for more than one hospital day after a woman gives birth under certain circumstances. Here again, active involvement by an informed public is needed. Health-care plans have severely limited coverage of mental-health treatment, compelling many mental-health professionals to seek other work. At the same time the plans may cover psychoactive medications such as Prozac, Zoloft, Lithium, and Haloperidol. Although these drugs are useful, they will never completely replace the need for psychotherapy, or talk therapy, despite the difficulty of proving that psychotherapy is "cost-effective."

We need to look at how research is paid for and who will be paid to do it. No longer do hospital-based practitioner-physicians carry out much of the present immense amount of research. It is almost impossible for a clinician, that is to say a practicing doctor, to carry out research involving the basic sciences. The M.D. degree alone is less and less sought after and less often a factor in the awarding of research grants, principally by the National Institutes of Health (NIH). The majority of the still well-funded grant money goes to full-time holders of the Ph.D. or Ph.D. and M.D. degrees. Basic science research, which is essential to progress, has almost eclipsed bedside "clinical" research, as has been well documented by Dr. Edward H. Ahrens Jr. of the Rockefeller University in his book *The Crisis in Clinical Research*. Observations made on actual patients, tabulated and analyzed, are the basis of clinical research, which should go hand in hand with basic science. Basic science research is totally separated from people with illnesses, and it takes place far from the bedside, in medical school, university, or pharmaceutical firms' laboratories. All of the spectacular medical advances of the last fifty years began in these laboratories.

The costs of our marvelously successful biomedical/medical school research should probably be separated from the money that is paid for direct medical care. This is a difficult task (but not impossible, as some people think). Corporate funding, for-profit, is one way to pay for part of the costs of basic science research, which we must continue at a very high level. However, this method will need close supervision. Privatization of research cannot fail in some cases to lead to projects biased toward the possibility of lucrative returns from the discovery of practical applications. The most basic scientific research is the foundation of all progress, and it will always need to be funded by governments. We cannot afford, as a nation, to fail to support basic science.

There is an irreducible minimum level of health care on which almost everyone should be able to agree. It is hard to live with the notion that at present 40 million Americans are uninsured and that such massive expenses as they may incur from cancer, heart disease, or through injuries in automobile accidents or as victims of violence, just to name a few examples, will have to come out of their own pocket or from the uncompensated care funds in hospitals. By putting off medical care as much and as long as possible, the uninsured are at greater risk of serious illness, which might have been prevented. This country really should be able to afford for everyone at the least to have access to emergency care and treatment, within limits to be determined, of life-threatening illnesses.

The path of least resistance to general health insurance up to this time has been to place the responsibility on the employer. We are now witnessing the catastrophic results of this popular policy.

Companies, looking at the costs of doing business, have discovered that they can save money on health-insurance premiums by laying off full-time employees. The work can still get done by part-time or contract workers—"temps" and others—and employers don't have to pay these workers' benefits. These uninsured workers shop around to try to find affordable health insurance. Meanwhile the insurers, for their part, have contracted with firms that employ large numbers of people who are well enough and young enough to work. This means that everyone else who is applying as an individual is in a higher-risk pool and must pay exorbitant rates for comprehensive coverage. As a result, many individuals do not have any coverage whatsoever or are grossly underinsured.

Can we have it all? Not unless we train many more caregivers to deliver the services that people want and at the same time lower the expectations of entitlements for every person. To continue to enjoy the fruits of our technological innovations, we must find a way to pay for them. We cannot have it all unless we achieve universal coverage, which is most likely to occur through a single-payer system, based on tax funds. All these wishes are not "pie in the sky," and achieving these goals will not happen in our lifetime. In the meantime, therefore, it is necessary for all of us to make the best plans possible in order not to be victims, and above all we all need to save for that rainy day that will surely come when we will not be covered by insurance. The quality of life itself is not reimbursable—that is up to each of us. In health and in sickness the outcome often depends on luck; luck that cannot be mandated, supplied by the government, or covered by insurance.

Good health is a privilege, but whether or not it is a right is debatable. It seems hard for many of us Americans to accept the fact that someday we will all get old, we will be ill, and someday we will all die. No health plan will ever alter these fundamental facts, so it is a waste of time to blame others for them. Illness or accident are inevitable sooner or later. It helps to recall that most illnesses are self-limited, that is, they are not fatal, and given time, the body will heal itself. Human beings are fundamentally tough.

One's well-being is dependent upon many positive factors such as feeling well, self-knowledge, having financial security, a stable family, and a congenial job with some job security. With some degree of certainty you can make things better for yourself in regard to your health, by such means as a healthy diet, regular exercise, abstention from unhealthy habits, and a positive outlook on life. Beyond that, good health depends on a long-term view of life that has higher goals and some purpose.

Taking care of yourself involves knowing yourself and knowing what you want, as well as knowing the health-care options available, with all of their inclusions and limitations. For instance, if you elect one of the alternative methods of care, under the present system, these services may not be covered by insurance plans, so you'll have to pay the whole cost.

Having said all these things, it is time to make decisions about what kind of health care and what kind of doctor you are going to seek. Life consists of difficult decisions made with incomplete information. No one will ever have all the facts available, but as an old saying has it, "If you don't know where you are going, you won't get there." The cornerstone of the best medical care is and always will be a good, mutually trusting doctor-patient relationship. With a lot of diligence and a little luck everyone someday, I hope, will achieve this goal.

2

Patients Today

*It is worthwhile to secure the happiness of the patient as
well as to prolong his life.*

WILLIAM J. MAYO

People today are worried sick, but not for fear of an epidemic or
some fatal illness. There seems to be a general feeling of uncertainty: about the country and where it is going, about job security
and the economy, and especially about their health and how to get
the health care they want at a price they can afford.

There is a difference between those suffering with serious illnesses (which they may or may not acknowledge) and those sometimes referred to as "the worried well." Among the population of
health-care consumers, it is hard to strike a balance between excessive concern over some symptoms and overlooking or intentionally
ignoring danger signs. More and more it is certain that people
should have more self-knowledge and more practical knowledge
of certain warning signals. It is as bad to be the macho denier of
symptoms as it is to be the person panicking over every variation

from normal, usual feeling. The trouble is that one can never be certain.

To put things in perspective, the health of most people is very good most of the time. Most illnesses and injuries are minor and heal on their own. Immunizations have greatly improved our statistics for morbidity (illness) and mortality. Even so, we are not the healthiest, nor the longest-living people in the world for a variety of reasons. Mostly for economic reasons the immunization rates for our children are almost the worst among the developed countries. Studies of managed-care plans have shown clearly that they achieve higher rates of immunization than do fee-for-service (indemnity) plans, not only for childhood diseases, but for tetanus, influenza, and pneumonia vaccinations for adults. This is a good example of enlightened self-interest, since because of diligence the plan will have to pay out less for caring for preventable illnesses. The time, trouble, and expense of going to a private fee-for-service physician is a powerful disincentive. Schools and boards of health in some states have also achieved high rates of immunization at relatively little cost.

Unfortunately, many of us tend to have bad habits that have a negative impact on health. We smoke a lot, use a lot of alcohol and drugs, and lead the world in the consumption of "junk food." More people have been killed or maimed in automobile accidents than all those who have been killed or injured in all the wars in which we have participated. These are all shortcomings or hazards that we can remedy if we try. At present the figures showing the millions of preventable deaths resulting from such factors are depressing.

Safe drinking water and proper sewage disposal have probably saved more lives than have doctors, and any success in the battles for eliminating the hazards of radiation, air pollution, and contaminated food products will save many more. These are not glamorous subjects, however, and we seem to prefer the fantasy that the modern medical miracles we see on television and read about in the press make a huge difference. Statistically speaking they do not.

Why, then, are people so health conscious and anxious? We emphasize health in schools; for fund-raising purposes we publicize the hazards of cancer, heart disease, diabetes, birth defects, multiple sclerosis, myasthenia, tuberculosis, venereal disease, AIDS, mental illness, and many other diseases and conditions. These are all real problems, but the sum total of the onslaught of threats of fearful diseases in the media produces at the very least anxieties about health. The drain on the health-care dollar owing to tests performed on the worried well is enormous, but who dares to say these people are not entitled to frequent testing and visits to the doctor? The healthy person who is afraid he or she may have cancer or AIDS or clogged coronary arteries suffers just as much before the proper examinations and tests are done as the one who has the disease. Hypochondriacs are well known to have just as much "real" illness as anyone else. Health-care professionals may have a hard time giving equal attention and a sympathetic hearing to a patient they suspect has no "real" organic disease. Deciding how far to pursue testing and questioning is an art as hard to develop as it is to define. Time to listen and to think is essential to developing this art.

More and more doctors are working on the system known as "capitation." The doctor is paid a fixed amount per head; the more patients on his or her panel, the more money comes in. Under capitation, the doctor loses money by taking too much time with any one patient. In addition, the patient who insists on further tests is in danger of becoming an adversary rather than an ally of the doctor. The patient quite naturally wants every assurance that all necessary test results are available. But ordering tests costs the doctor money, either directly or through penalties imposed by the managed-care firm employing him. Cutting down on unnecessary testing may be a praiseworthy way of reducing health-care costs, but patients may begin to question the doctor's commitment to offering the best care.

Without looking for trouble, the patient needs to know what might happen if something goes wrong while he or she is a member of the plan. That is, the mechanisms for conflict management, grievance procedures, appeals from denials of service, and mechanisms available for switching from one primary-care doctor to another if necessary.

Some other features of our country today add to people's anxiety about health. One is the cult of youthfulness, exaggerated in the United States to a degree not seen in other countries. Face lifts, hair transplants, liposuction, and hormone injections are expensive weapons in the always-losing battle against aging. Plastic surgery and restorative dentistry often help people, but whether these should be paid for in all cases by health insurance or by the patients themselves is debatable. The solution, if any, is not medical or economic, but social.

Long-term health problems can be devastating. Such problems as facial defects, childhood abuse, hearing and vision disabilities, and physical and developmental disabilities, such as mental retardation and cerebral palsy, need to be identified and treated as early as possible to give people the chance to lead more productive and satisfying lives. Treatment may be long-term and costly. Insurers should not impose spending caps for such conditions or refuse to cover them as "preexisting conditions."

Psychotherapy for problems involving personal identity and interpersonal relations is extremely important to many Americans, but it is very expensive. Who should pay, and how, is a test of our national will and of our degree of concern for others. Some would argue that health-care reform financing should be all inclusive, because separating social concerns from medical is problematic. If a psychological problem causes the loss of a job, failure in school or college, the disintegration of a marriage, or the abuse of children, a plan, to be considered truly comprehensive, should pay for part or all of the treatment, because these are to some extent outcomes measurable in dollars. Pharmacotherapy (the prescription of psychoactive drugs such as Prozac) can never replace the mental-health professional's work of listening and counseling, but it may be needed as a supplement. At the other end of the scale, no health plan can afford to pay for repairs to everyone's self-image or to help sort out intrafamily adjustment problems. Finding the middle ground is remarkably difficult. Substance abuse and addiction have a measurable dollar cost, so treatment must either be covered by a health plan or a separately funded government source.

Putting together the facts contributing to your own good health is the best way to get to know yourself and your potential health-care needs. The predispositions you inherit from your parents and other ancestors are factors you cannot at this time change (perhaps someday this will change). You can change your risks for developing certain health conditions, such as high blood pressure, coronary artery disease, cancer, and stroke by reducing stress, eating a balanced, healthy diet, exercising regularly, drinking only in moderation, and giving up smoking.

Going to the Doctor

When you do go to a doctor (or hospital or medical clinic) it means that you are looking for help, which you deserve. This experience is an unpleasant one for almost everyone. It involves some loss of autonomy, the feeling that you have lost control over what is happening to you. You have a feeling of nervousness, even a feeling of fear of impending spiritual and physical exposure. This brings out defensive feelings and sometimes as an unfortunate result people tend to conceal some facts essential to the proper diagnosis and treatment of a particular complaint. Women, through past experience, are very often afraid that they will be "put down" or treated as second-class helpless people. The male ego is often connected with projecting an image of invulnerability and correctness, so men often have a deep fear that they will be exposed. Everyone should try to avoid these pitfalls by being honest and open with the doctor.

Sometimes scientifically correct diagnosis and treatment is not the patient's immediate concern. The Gospel according to St. Matthew puts it this way: "Is there anyone among you, if your child asks for bread, will give a stone?" Nowhere is this more deeply felt than with the fear or pain (or both) that brings you, the patient, into the doctor's office, looking for help.

In most cases, you have decided that you *should* go to see your doctor, not that you *want* to do so. Besides costing money and time, the prospect brings up memories of past illnesses, pains, fears, and embarrassments. You would probably like to put off the visit, but a friend or loved one has persuaded you to go. You know from past experience that dropping in without an appointment will involve at the least a long wait, and at the worst you will find that you cannot be seen that day because the problem does not rise to the level of an emergency. Therefore, you have to telephone first.

In a large group or clinic practice your call will be directed to an appointment secretary, who tries to guess how much time to set aside and how urgent the request is. After some discussion and persuasion, you are given an appointment. Given the busy practice of a physician with limited office hours, you may have to wait weeks or even months. Now you see why we need more rather than fewer primary-care doctors, along with a better system of sorting out health-care needs and a system for delivering prompt care. Doctors in private offices and in smaller communities usually see patients more promptly than do city specialists, especially those attached to a teaching hospital. If enough patients have bombarded your doctor's secretary with urgent pleas, the result is that more names are "squeezed in" the schedule resulting in longer waits and a less relaxed doctor.

You go to the office and announce your presence. When you arrive for your doctor's appointment, almost everywhere now and certainly everywhere in the future, you will be required to produce an identification card and to fill out and sign a registration form. You are then entered into the computer system and can proceed to the next step, which is to sit in the waiting room until it is your turn.

It is natural to feel self-conscious in the waiting room. You try not to stare at other people. With luck, you will be politely greeted. Ideally the waiting room should be large enough to have more than enough seats at all times. Seats should be arranged so that one needn't stare into someone else's face, but this seldom seems to be the case. A waiting room that is not spotlessly clean makes a poor impression.

Soon your name is called. It is your turn. By now everybody knows your identity, and you may wish that you had been called by number, rather than by name. You are ushered into the consulting-room office, or in a busy practice, sometimes directly to the examination room, before you see the doctor. You make your customary greeting as does the doctor, and the interview begins with the doctor asking what is wrong. (A few years ago two medical sociologists taped, with permission, many doctor-patient interviews. In a majority of instances, the patient's opening statement was interrupted by the doctor in the first sentence.) You persist in trying to give an objective account. The doctor asks relevant questions, which are intended to be open-ended, but often he or she unconsciously directs the response.

The first visit is often a strain on both parties; the real fears and facts often do not emerge until a second or third visit, unless the doctor is able to offer you thirty minutes, more or less, of sympathetic listening. At the first interview, both patient and doctor may want to avoid embarrassing topics, even though these may be at the core of the patient's complaints. These include unusual sexual feelings or practices, sexual or spousal abuse, verbal or physical assault, unwanted pregnancy, dissatisfaction with size of one's body parts, bad breath, abortion, contraception, and the inevitable consequences of aging.

Now it is time for the examination. You may be asked to take off all or most of your clothes, even before the doctor and you have discussed the necessity for it. The reason for these seemingly unfeeling maneuvers is simply the pressure of time. If the doctor's assistant can help carry out a system in which there are patients in two different examining rooms and the present complaint has been written down on a chart, the doctor can then go rapidly from one patient to another, saving time and increasing productivity. What such a system does to the doctor-patient relationship should be obvious. When the doctor must leave the examining room to answer an urgent call, the minutes seem like hours to the partly naked, shivering patient.

Sometimes the encounter between doctor and patient consists only of talk, which is quite often, under the circumstances, all that is required or desired. Many patients, though, want more tangible evidence of contact. A visit even for something as simple as a head cold or a sore throat should involve the actual "laying on of hands" and inspection. No matter how sure your doctor may be of the diagnosis, the ritual of the physical examination, partial or complete, must take place. If you are given a prescription or laboratory requisition without having received any "laying on of hands," you may feel cheated. Naturally, the unclothed body yields the most information. Both your doctor and you may be inclined to minimize the undressing to save time and to avoid excessive invasion of privacy, but you deserve the examination, so you should not resist disrobing to the extent required. It takes a bit more time to listen to the heart and lungs and to take the blood pressure of a patient who comes in with what appears to be a minor respiratory infection, but this ritual not only protects the physician from an accusation of impersonal superficiality, but gives the patient a sense of closeness and caring. Furthermore, sometimes an important, unexpected physical finding appears in the process. And a diagnosis may, in fact, be missed altogether by the omission of a full examination.

This ritual, of course, often demands the presence of a chaperone, if doctor and patient are of different gender and the examination is an intimate one. Risk-management guidelines of many HMOs are quite specific on this point. Most medical schools give sensitivity training to both male and female students in their first and second years about the proper procedures and decorum of the physical examination.

When you and your doctor have known each other for some time, after several visits, the examination ritual becomes simpler, quicker, and less emotionally charged. The doctor and nurse will know you better and will know what to expect from you; and you will know what to expect of them. You notice that the doctor always washes his or her hands. You know what to expect from the examination. You hope it is as brief as possible, while not omitting any important, relevant details.

Soon the examination is completed, often all too soon, and you are told to get dressed and are handed a prescription or two, or perhaps a requisition to take to the laboratory for testing. It is often at this stage of the encounter between doctor and patient that the symptom or thought that is really bothering the patient comes out. Every physician is familiar with the patient who, with one hand on the doorknob apparently about to leave, says, "Oh, just one more thing, Doctor," and then delivers perhaps in an embarrassed monotone an emotionally charged revelation. At this point no matter how pressed for time and how aware the doctor is of the other patients in the waiting room, the doctor must exercise great restraint by asking the patient to sit down and to explain further the matter that is bothering him or her.

Many times the parting words of the doctor may be hurried, and you may also want to get out of the examining room as soon as possible. Resist the temptation to leave in a hurry. Verbal instructions and conclusions at this point are often forgotten. You should always write down what the doctor tells you before you leave, and ask any questions you need to ask to understand what has come up during the visit. Lack of even the simplest sort of explanation of the medical situation brings panic closer. The next step, be it further testing or a return visit, referral, or prescription, must be clear in your mind before you leave.

Having made these assessments, you can at leisure, at home, consider whether this is the health-care provider you want, be it nurse, physician, or alternative therapist. This is the time to consult your impressions of the caregiver. Did he or she maintain eye contact? Was his or her manner professional yet caring? Did he or she take the time to answer your questions? It is easier to change doctors sooner rather than later.

Both patients and health-care providers are happier when there is a functioning appointment system. Under the best of circumstances, the delay for a follow-up appointment should be minimal. A long wait is hard on the patient and sometimes even dangerous. Patients can and should be treated as promptly as safety permits, often before a definitive diagnosis can be achieved. Fear becomes much less gripping when the patient can be assured that a friendly, firm, confident person has determined a plan of action. Every delay, even if it is inevitable, compounds the pain or fear.

At the same time, the conscientious physician, knowing that there are people who have been waiting a long time, feels anxious and hurried. Unfortunately, the duration and severity of illnesses are not always predictable, so that emergencies may interrupt. If you plead with the appointment secretary to "just squeeze me in somewhere, I don't mind," the result is overbooking, long waits, and hurried consultations. The more successful and highly regarded a physician, the more difficult it is to obtain an appointment in the near future. On the other hand, any clinical practice or managed-care system that constantly saddles its practitioners with a load of patients who cannot be handled adequately in a reasonable period of time will get a bad reputation among patients.

Many clinics and hospitals have a walk-in center for the non-emergency care of matters that will not take a great deal of time. This, of course, means that at each visit you are apt to see a different doctor, who must take time to become acquainted with your previous medical history. To make the visit go more smoothly, arm yourself with as many facts as you can get about the way the system functions, bring with you as much information as you can about your medical history, and be courteous with the person who makes the appointment. These principles apply even more so to emergency room visits, discussed in chapter 7.

At a walk-in center, the clerk who receives the patient, the nurse in charge of the office or clinic, and the doctor frequently forget that you come into such clinics feeling vulnerable, defenseless, and needy. The patient's vulnerable state gives a power to the physician and nurse that should never be used for personal advantage or bullying. As a patient, you may be a rather private person and not at ease with strangers, so you'll want to feel sure that your privacy will be respected, that your concerns are taken seriously, and that any open admissions you make about lifestyle or attitudes will be treated with respect. At this time a little friendly conversation and courteous treatment go a long way toward establishing mutual trust and sense of caring; a "new contract" for patients and doctors needs to have such considerations as a cornerstone.

Taking children to the doctor or clinic can be a good or a bad experience, as every parent knows. Past experience, a friendly and caring receptionist and nurse, and a friendly and attentive doctor can make this an easy and productive visit. Many pediatric group practices, in or out of managed care, have handouts explaining policies and procedures to try to make the visit as smooth as possible. The visit can also be made easier if the parent or parents try to bring in the child with an air of affection and confidence, often despite their own fears or anxiety. This is more easily said than done. A child can sense the feelings of parents toward their own medical caregivers and the system. A child needs to feel that going to the doctor is not a punishment and that both parents like and trust the nurse and doctor. The pressure on the staff to deal with a full waiting room, with one eye on the clock and the other on the appointment schedule, may make it difficult for parents and caregivers always to appear calm and cheerful.

The child who has a positive feeling for the pediatrician and nurse will have an easier time coping with his or her own health problems as an adult. But try as we may, we cannot always be sure of what the child thinks and feels about the visit to the doctor. Early in my practice, one child said to his mother: "I like Dr. Prout, but his stethoscope is cold, and Dr. Kimball's is warm."

The Doctor-Patient Relationship

Sometimes in the urgent press of patients and their demands, it is hard for caregivers to remember to be, first of all, people who care and who are there to relieve suffering. At the same time the patient is, of course, absorbed in his or her own problem and may not be aware of the stresses in the office or clinic, and may act out in a defensive manner that can hinder communication. In such cases it is best to keep in mind that by keeping the interchange positive you are more apt to have a good outcome. If the doctor says in a brusque and impersonal way, "Well, what seems to be the matter with you?" and you reply, "Well, that's what I'm paying you to find out," roadblocks have been set up. When the same encounter starts with the doctor saying, "Hello — — —, I see that you seem to be in some pain. What seems to be the matter?" and then if you reply with a simple statement of what is bothering you, then the right diagnosis is apt to be made sooner, and treatment can be started to relieve not only the underlying cause but the symptoms that brought you there in the first place.

Earlier I quoted one patient who felt that the doctor was too close and personal, and another who felt that the same doctor was too impersonal. The doctor-patient relationship works best when both parties proceed cautiously and politely. The proper balance of closeness can only be achieved gradually, and with mutual motivation to make it work, as doctor and patient get to know each other. Admittedly, this is the ideal. The pressure of limited allotted time may lead both patient and doctor to cut short the amenities, sometimes with unfortunate results. In many practices patients are more comfortable with the nurse practitioner or other assistant and rarely feel the need to communicate with their doctor. This arrangement can be satisfactory to everyone, particularly the business manager, because the nurse is paid less than the physician.

One of the chief complaints of American patients is that doctors do not listen to them. By the same token, many doctors become impatient with what appears to be irrelevant or unnecessary social conversation on the part of patients. The tactful assistant or nurse who is sympathetic and listens is of enormous benefit to both patient and doctor at this point. The patient feels that there is a caring and sympathetic team, an extension of the doctor. The assistant is an extra pair of eyes and ears supplying the needed information to the doctor.

Doctors and patients may come from different cultures and customs, and this may create a barrier in their relationship. For example, a patient's feelings about undressing in front of a stranger or someone of the opposite sex without a chaperone standing by are important considerations. The fear of loss of modesty keeps many older women and men who have perhaps come from a more cloistered culture and background from going to the doctor at all. It is for this reason that schools of medicine and nursing are trying to instruct students in the variations of cultures and customs and attitudes in our heterogeneous nation. For example, Hispanic men often insist on being beside their wives or daughters at all times, especially in the presence of a male doctor. Muslims are particularly sensitive to meticulous hand-washing by the medical team. Some Muslims even feel that the left hand is to be used only in toilet functions and should not touch the patient even after hand-washing. Scandinavians are often more reticent about discussing their feelings, especially sexual feelings, than people from warmer climates. Loyalty to the family and family honor supersedes all considerations to many people of Greek or Italian origin, so that the existence of sexually transmitted disease, substance abuse, or family violence may be concealed. Some people wish to have physicians only of their own race or religion. The choice of a physician within their health plan may be limited, setting up a barrier to good doctor-patient relations.

Many women have been socialized not to speak up and demand what they want. By the same token, women who have learned to speak up are sometimes labeled as excessively aggressive and treated accordingly. For men, the situation is somewhat different. Men are socialized to be macho, not to admit weakness; therefore, they are slow to recognize their own problems and to seek help. Men are frequently afraid of having some weakness exposed and may need to change to a physician who is sympathetic, nonjudgmental, and who takes time to hear the fears behind the stated complaints. In another highly sensitive field, children and adolescents are reluctant to speak out about sexual abuse, in the family or out of it, and women are notorious for being reluctant to mention spousal abuse. Identifying all of these factors depends on mutual trust and forbearance.

Some conditions and diagnoses are as frustrating and stressful for the doctor as they are for the patient and the family, in particular those for which the doctor can offer little or no hope. For example, some types of cancer are mostly incurable, and AIDS at present is apparently always a fatal disease. Chronic-fatigue syndrome is hard to define precisely, is persistent, and is baffling to treat. People hope, of course, for a magic cure, or at least relief. Patients' expectations of cure and their subsequent disappointment may sometimes bring them to doubt the doctor's competence. The competence of the renowned, altogether admirable Centers for Disease Control in Atlanta was called into doubt when Legionnaires' disease was first identified. One congressman called for the removal of the director of the CDC shortly afterward because he had not immediately found a cause and a cure. As it turned out, the cause, the epidemiology, and the proper treatment were identified in record time. As far as I know, no public apology for this congressman's attack was forthcoming.

All of us who are doctors share the experience of trying to give hope and comfort when the diagnosis is elusive, and there is no satisfactory treatment. Understandably, patients will be frustrated in such situations. Sometimes it appears that one way out is for the doctor to succumb to the urge to pass the patient along to another specialist, or to embark on a new series of tests, rather than to spend hours searching for an answer that may never come, or worse yet, to say bluntly that there is no hope, that nothing can be done. It takes skill, experience, and courage for the caring doctor to admit defeat. Patients might want to keep in mind that doctors don't have all the answers and cannot always provide a cure.

Patients want caring, time, and thoroughness. Doctors and nurses want to provide these elements of care, but the pressures and regulations of the money people are a powerful disincentive. Patients and doctors have the same objectives and are natural allies. They have everything to gain by resisting the trend to further depersonalize and commercialize the essential need for the relief of suffering.

3

Caregivers

*There are no members of society whose pursuits lead them
to listen more frequently to what has been exquisitely
termed the still sad music of humanity.*

Samuel Warren

Doctors

No matter how medical systems have changed and will continue to
change, the central figure in patient care will always be a doctor.
Nevertheless, doctors and patients will be working increasingly
with nurses, other doctors, administrators, technicians, case workers, and others. Doctors have held a high status socially and eco-
nomically, but their place is rapidly changing. More of the public is
knowledgeable, especially in health-care matters. People in general
are pleased with the advances in medical knowledge and technology, but many are of two minds about doctors of medicine. Re-
peated references to the high income of physicians is one factor,
and public airing of malpractice actions is another. Unfortunately,

the good deeds and caring work of the majority of doctors are not newsworthy.

TRENDS IN THE MEDICAL PROFESSION

Most doctors enter the profession with high hopes of an exciting and rewarding career. After years of talking at length with many hundreds of premedical and medical students, I continue to be impressed by the consistency of their goals. They want to have an intellectually stimulating occupation, with good financial standing to be sure, but always with a degree of wanting to be useful to other people. Many want the satisfaction of a mutually trusting, friendly relationship with patients. Very few nowadays begin by wanting or expecting to get rich. This outlook is realistic; changes in the health-care system make it very unlikely that doctors will become rich in the future.

Under managed care, the primary-care doctors will do more of the work formerly carried out by specialists. Specialists, whose numbers exceed the need for them, will have to accept sharply reduced salaries from the health-plan managers. No matter how devoted to their profession and proud of the special capacity to help, specialists' attitudes toward money may become affected by such factors as heavy indebtedness and the desire to keep up with or exceed the income of their peers.

There are too many surgeons at present in this country according to manpower studies and managed-care statistics, although their distribution is uneven; there are too many in the cities and too few in rural areas. Residencies in surgical training have already been reduced by as much as 20 percent. The competition for the more coveted surgical programs is intense. Forty years ago, very few women and even fewer minority students were able to receive the training to become board-certified surgeons. This imbalance is being redressed now, but they and all other would-be surgeons face greater obstacles on the way to their goal.

In the 1970s and 1980s the number of Americans applying to medical schools fell to such a degree that admission became much less selective and was a source of worry to medical educators. This has changed in the last three years. Medical-school applications are now at an all-time high, and there is more hope than ever that our future doctors will not merely be the brightest but the best people. There are probably many reasons behind this unexpected and sharp increase in the number of premedical students. Disillusionment among college students with the worlds of business and finance, and overcrowding of the legal profession, compounded by the shrinkage in white-collar jobs in industry may be partly responsible.

Despite the expressed unhappiness of older practicing physicians, and the much-publicized drawbacks of working in a managed-care setting, these thousands of well-qualified young applicants have not yet been turned off, so they give us hope for the future. The pool of entering students increasingly reflects diversity of gender, race, and socioeconomic strata. The number of doctors of medicine in active practice rose from 311,000 in 1970 to 606,000 in 1992, according to the *Statistical Abstract of the United States*. The greater part of this increase came from the increase in the number of specialists.

The stereotype of the doctor as a white male is in retreat. For example, the classes of 1998 and 1999 at Harvard Medical School, formerly an almost all white male school, have a majority of women; white males make up only 30 percent of these classes. Almost every medical school now makes a conscientious effort not only to accept minority applicants, but to recruit them actively. We can expect that patients more and more will be able to have physicians with whom they feel at ease, as diversity and social mixing increase in the profession.

More and more physicians are women. Temperamentally, women

are generally more sympathetic and patient, but gender is no guarantee of these traits. Medical-school admissions interviewers report that women applicants are better listeners. Women usually prefer other women as gynecologists, but here again, patients vary, and some women actually prefer an authoritarian and paternalistic male doctor.

What It Takes to Be a Doctor

Selecting the "best" candidate from the large pool of qualified applicants is a major task of medical schools. The Association of American Medical Colleges (AAMC) has for many years studied the selection process and all its complexities. Some characteristics are obviously desirable: brains, scientific ability and training, and skill in problem solving, as well as a proven record of accomplishment. Racial, ethnic, and social diversity are increasingly considered. Less obvious but equally important is the need for above-average energy, a capacity for hard work in the face of discouragement, and stamina. But the traits we most want in a doctor are extremely hard to measure.

Many years ago Dr. Samuel Levine, a great pioneer cardiologist and a fine human being, was talking with a small group of medical students under my charge at the time about the practice of medicine. He asked them, "What is the first characteristic of a good physician?" Some suggested brains; others said hard work, originality, and other compelling virtues. "No," he said, "the most important trait a doctor can have is generosity." This capacity cannot be measured by testing or grading but only through experience. The patient can only sense it.

Integrity also can only be judged indirectly, and by long and close observation. It is another necessary trait in a physician, whose work is seldom directly observed at first hand and whose opinions and statements must be trusted. The physician must be honest with him- or herself as well as with the patient. Integrity is established early in life by example, by discipline, and by belief. Flagrant examples of dishonesty may be apparent in young people, and almost always occur more than once, forming a pattern that is usually noticed. Less obvious signs of lack of integrity are unfortunately often not reported. No medical-school applicant asks for a recommending letter from someone who does not trust him or her, so the value of letters of recommendation is less and less accepted in these days of litigation, worries about confidentiality, and political correctness.

After an extensive course of academic requirements in college, students embark usually on four years of medical school. Roughly, half of this education is in purely scientific studies—biomedical science of increasingly complex nature. The training in schools of osteopathy, leading to the D.O. degree, is similar. The other half of medical-school training consists of being introduced to and experiencing in some depth the care of patients under faculty supervision. Traditionally "bedside" teaching has been carried out in a large urban hospital associated with the medical school, usually using public "ward" patients as opposed to private patients. Medicaid, Medicare, and insurance plans have largely erased this distinction; the patients with whom medical students now work are not for the most part objects of charity, and they have the option of declining to be used as teaching subjects. As a result, the patients are treated with greater respect by students who are properly supervised. These days students learn to do such intrusive procedures as rectal and vaginal examinations, not on patients, but increasingly with paid models and using various "virtual reality" simulations.

At the same time, medical educators actively encourage the development of sensitivity to the feelings of both the patient and the student. Increasingly, medical schools have obligatory courses in ethics, sensitivity training, and social values. Further, more and more medical schools now require courses in literature as part of the standard curriculum. These consist of readings and discussions of works about life and death, suffering, and doctoring. The goal is to help the student to understand people and thereby to see how illness appears to the patient. In these courses, medical as well as nonmedical writings, plays, poems, novels, and biographies are used; they are a vivid way of teaching. Students learn to appreciate how people feel about doctors and medical care and perhaps can get in touch with their own reactions to illness, suffering, and death. The eminent and beloved researcher-physician-teacher Tinsley Harrison put it this way: "The true physician has a Shakespearean breadth of interest in the wise and foolish, the proud and the humble, the stoic hero and the whining rogue: He cares for people."

The powers of observation are critical to the development of clinical skills, but they must be coupled with reflection. Some teachers have their students read the Sherlock Holmes stories for the lessons they teach. In addition to observing and mentally recording everyday occurrences and behaviors, new doctors must learn to be curious: why do these things happen, and what do they mean? Sherlock Holmes in one case pointed out that when a certain dog did not bark, it was a significant variation, because the circumstances called for barking. Illness often comes in unexpected places, at unexpected times, requiring that the doctor always have his or her antennae up. Every doctor has had the experience at one time or another of overlooking a clue that was in plain sight, because the expectation of a significant finding was very low. When a school doctor sees hundreds of healthy students, his or her clinical alertness, known in the profession as the index of suspicion, can easily become dulled.

Even the experts may miss the obvious if they are not looking for it. In one of the clinical-research divisions of the National Institutes of Health in Washington, D.C., there is a self-service cafeteria, where every day hundreds of endocrine experts would bring their trays to a certain cashier, who had been working there for a long time. No one had commented on her appearance until one day, a visiting doctor asked his NIH companion, a distinguished expert on thyroid disorders, "How long has that woman had myxedema?"

This condition involves a total deficiency of thyroid hormone, and it produces a typical facial appearance. None of the resident experts had picked up on this, and they were chagrined. They had not been looking at a patient; they were looking (if at all) at a cashier.

Communication between caregivers and patients is critically important and needs to be emphasized continuously throughout medical school and residency training. For example, nurses and doctors out of habit and for reasons of efficiency and precision use medical terms that are often not understood by the patient. (As a patient, if you don't understand what the doctor says, speak up. Otherwise the doctor or nurse may think you have comprehended an order or an explanation, and will expect you to act accordingly.) Likewise, professionals need to be prepared for the peculiarities of speech or vocabulary of their patients—hence the need for a broadly multicultural staff and educational programs. There was a notorious instance of a misunderstanding years ago at a large teaching hospital. A woman who came from a Caribbean culture appeared at the reception desk of the eye clinic. The clerk asked her what was wrong with her vision, and she replied that there was nothing wrong, but that the admitting nurse in the emergency room had directed her to the eye clinic. When the matter was finally straightened out, it appeared that the patient had said to the emergency admitting nurse: "I haven't seen anything for three months." In her vernacular, this meant that she had not menstruated for three months. Finally she was correctly directed to the obstetrical unit.

As they proceed through their four years of medical school, students begin to select their choice of career. At every medical school there are printed guidelines available that try to introduce students to their options. One pharmaceutical firm has organized a widely used intensive program to assist medical students in the choice of careers. Over the years it has been my observation, however, that among students the influence of their peers and the careers of their own teachers are stronger factors.

With the typical American medical student who is heavily in debt and hoping to start a family, the pressure to make money in a hurry is hard to resist. Debts ranging from $50,000 to over $100,000 must be repaid after students complete residency training. Several studies reported to the Association of American Medical Colleges show that more and more young doctors put "lifestyle" at the top of their wish list. This means a guaranteed income, living in a desirable community, and having enough free time for a good social and family life. Medical schools need early and often to inform medical students of the realities that they won't get rich, and that they may have a limited choice of place where they can both live and practice. Under managed care it will no longer be possible for them to make a very large amount of money, although without any doubt highly skilled subspecialists such as cardiac surgeons, ophthalmological surgeons, and transplantation specialists will continue to be paid better than primary-care internists, primary care being defined as either family practice, general internal medicine, or general pediatrics. Because all health-care plans, as we will discuss, depend on an increasing number of primary-care physicians who will be generalists and will do much of the work now being referred to specialists, it is clear that students choosing primary care will expect to be paid much more than today's generalists. However, both primary-care doctors and specialists will earn less than they have in the past decades. As a result, the difference between the pay of generalists and specialists will no longer be such a powerful incentive to specialize. In Norway, for example, generalists are already paid more than specialists.

There are other factors that help shape young doctors as they proceed through medical school and residency training. Since fatigue is an almost constant companion, the energetic, strong man or woman will endure and perform better. The pressure to get patients' work-ups completed and to get the long waiting lines in the clinic disposed of brings an incentive to shorten the time spent with the patient and perhaps to cut corners. In the competition to get the best residency spots and after that the best training fellowships, the young doctor-in-training is tempted to imitate the instructors, professors, and successful department chiefs, taking on perhaps some of their less-desirable traits, along with their more desirable ones. The traditional framework of ethical behavior by doctors is not always consistent, because of what has been described as the medical profession's autonomous professional culture, which undervalues the patient's involvement in decision making and reinforces benign paternalism. These attitudes are obviously under attack and will undoubtedly change for the better.

Another force shaping the character and behavior of the doctor is the result of social pressures: racial friction, upward social mobility, and a sense of one's own identity and self-worth.

What to Expect from Your Doctor

What sort of people are doctors? All kinds, really, despite appearances and popular assumptions. Some are introverts, quiet people who do not communicate well with patients but who have superb medical knowledge and technical skills. Over time many of their patients appreciate these virtues and become devoted followers, but other patients move on. A larger number of doctors are more extroverted and communicative, but they vary in other ways.

It helps you, the patient, if you know what approach a given doctor will take with you. In a general way, surgeons and surgical specialists, such as orthopedists and ophthalmologists, want to size up the medical problem as rapidly as possible, make a decision, and act on it, which in most cases is the correct solution for the problems they encounter.

With surgery, the dramatic side of the work is obvious. It is the stuff on which movies and television series thrive. In reality, being in the operating room takes up only a part of the surgeon's time. For a surgeon, it is the brains, the training, and the ability to make decisions quickly, on the basis of such evidence as may be available, that are far more important than the operative manual skills. In general, surgeons like best to attack a definite problem, with a plan resulting in prompt action. The interpersonal side of the doctor-patient relationship is not of the greatest interest to them. A prolonged period of follow-up, which may include becoming involved in the patient's daily living, is alien to the temperament of many surgeons, desirable as it may be. I in no way mean to suggest that surgeons are not compassionate, because for the most part they are. Their desire to be healers may at times be coupled with some impatience with a disease process that is slow to comprehend, ambiguous, and uncertain of outcome. In such cases the primary-care doctor or nurse fills a useful role.

Surgical temperament is often well suited to clinical research. Many surgeons in the latter half of the twentieth century have made outstanding contributions to medicine. For example, Dr. Evarts Graham, over fifty years ago in St. Louis, pioneered in open-chest surgery and was one of the first to associate smoking with lung cancer. His work was based on basic research on the physiology of breathing and circulation. Dr. Francis D. Moore of Boston, as a relatively young man, published a landmark book based on the research coming from his and other laboratories, and those of many other basic scientists, which described in detail the bodily changes during and after surgery. Many lives have been saved by these now universally applied principles of surgical care. Three surgeons in Boston working together with internists and basic scientists brought about the first successful human transplant (of a kidney), opening up an entirely new field and saving or prolonging countless lives.

Dr. Harvey Cushing, outstanding as a U.S. Army surgeon in World War I, and later one of the founding fathers of neurosurgery, epitomized the need for a surgeon to be knowledgeable, to be prepared, and to be decisive, but careful, when he said, "A man can bleed to death from a severed carotid artery in a minute; you can save his life if you do not hurry."

Neurologists and psychiatrists, in general (and there are, of course, always exceptions), like to take time, to consider many facets of the case, and perhaps to defer any active decision making. Family practitioners and general internists fall in between. The advantage of having a personal primary-care doctor who knows you is that he or she can steer you in the right direction. However, in some cases you may have to be quite insistent to get an appointment with the specialist you want.

As we have said, pain is commonly what brings people to the doctor. All of us are uncomfortable witnessing others in pain, and doctors are no exception. It is less uncomfortable if they overlook, minimize, or even deny the existence of a patient's pain. But the sufferer senses the avoidance by doctors or nurses and becomes even more anxious. The true healer acknowledges the patient's pain and does not shrink from facing it with the patient. This takes insight and maturity, which are capacities that cannot be taught in a laboratory or classroom.

In chapter 1, some people were quoted who felt that their doctors were condescending or dictatorial; others felt that the doctor was either too remote or too close. These attitudes and feelings obviously occur in other life situations, but in the doctor-patient relationship, they are a real barrier to the open exchange of sensitive information the doctor needs to make a diagnosis, and they also leave the patient vulnerable. Condescension is usually unintended; the doctor who behaves this way may be lacking in professional and social self-confidence, and may feel the need to assume a superior position with patients. We can only hope that with continuing improvements in the selection and education of medical students that more physicians will become self-aware.

Your doctor needs your respect and confidence, but he or she at the same time needs to be prepared to describe the thinking behind the diagnosis and treatment, often to debate it with a well-informed patient. A clash of egos may result. In addition, the patient may understandably fear that a profit-driven, finance-oriented system is influencing the doctor's actions. This is a very realistic fear for many people. The doctor-patient relationship is delicate and needs nurturing. It is hard to imagine how this can happen in a managed-care interview limited to ten minutes, unless the patient and the physician have been fortunate enough to know each other well from past contacts.

PUT YOURSELF IN THE DOCTOR'S SHOES

The traditional role of the physician as the boss, in whom complete faith existed, goes far back in history, long before modern scientific medicine. In the past there were few effective treatments, but faith accomplished much. Also, most illnesses and injuries eventually heal of their own accord. Many treatments were of a sort of faith healing, what is now called the placebo effect. (A placebo is a totally inactive substance given to the patient intentionally along with strong assurance that it will be effective.) The skilled, old-time conscientious practitioner generally wished to help the patient but did not deceive himself. The quack was often just as effective then as now, because of the tendency for sick people's bodies to get well of their own accord. Most illnesses that cause fear and suffering respond to sympathy, suggestion, and reassurance.

Also, historically, the physician (along with the lawyer, the clergyman, and the teacher) was educated, and his patients were not. The physician could speak with an authority that was seldom contradicted. Molière in France and Ben Jonson in England lampooned the self-important dogmatism of doctors. In some respects things did not change much in the next three hundred years. Now patients are educated and are constantly bombarded with medical information. They expect answers to all their questions. The relationship under these circumstances is bound to change.

In order to understand the behavior of your doctor it might help to be familiar with some of the pressures he or she faces. The training period is longer. The indebtedness is greater. The exponential increase of scientific knowledge must be somehow, to the greatest extent possible, incorporated into practice. The physician is losing autonomy under managed care; we are witnessing the Götterdämmerung of the private physician. There is increased pressure on your generalist to take care of every complaint and not refer any to a specialist. Your generalist is aware of the possibility of being penalized for doing too much in the way of testing, or for hospitalizing too many people. At the same time, fears of malpractice actions create pressure not to omit important tests. The doctor, therefore, is confronted with a double whammy. After the case is closed, a deskbound reviewer assesses it and may judge that a normal test result indicates unnecessary caution, or that a potentially useful test could have been done, and the failure to order it is an omission. There often comes a time when tests do not reveal the answer, and judgment, partly intuitive, comes into play. A later reviewer may second-guess the doctor because the reviewer knows the outcome. Hospitalization is one way the generalist can respond to pressure from the family and to uncertainty in diagnosis. Increasingly the requirements of HMOs and other kinds of managed care call for the briefest possible doctor-patient encounter, which is frustrating to both parties. When the physician is restricted to five, ten, or fifteen minutes for the interview, the danger is that while establishing the first outlines of the complaint, the patient's real concerns may not emerge. Even if all the patient's concerns are aired, the physician may have great difficulty ascertaining the real problem and knowing how to advise the patient. The doctor in a hurry does not want to miss anything that might be turned up by a test, and as a result the doctor is more likely to overtest and overprescribe. The public and medical profession each have a stake in attempting to improve this sort of impersonal transaction, but more time, adequately financed, will not come cheap.

Every doctor feels pressure to keep up with new developments. Lifelong learning is an imperative for the medical profession. Scientific advances are constant; basic science discoveries are constantly being implemented, and new diagnostic and treatment methods come into practice very rapidly. For example, from the identification of the mysteries of DNA in the 1960s to the practical application of such knowledge in the treatment of a large number of disease processes took less than a decade. Continuing medical education is a requirement for doctors as well as for nurses. Many specialties require a recertification examination after several years, to assure up-to-date practices. Studying for examinations, doctors and nurses find, does not end at graduation. In a busy and fatiguing practice, to take time out for study at home, or in postgraduate courses, is a fact of life and one more added stress.

Doctors also need to take steps to inform their patients of the latest research findings as they relate to a given medical condition. In March 1996 Dr. W. A. Hensel wrote to the editor of the *New England Journal of Medicine* in response to an article recommending that before doing any PSA (prostate specific antigen) test for prostate cancer, the doctor should take the time to explain fully the PSA controversy to the patient. Even if the physician knows the up-to-the-minute status of this controversial issue, is he or she allowed by the health-care plan to take the ten or fifteen minutes to explain this one issue? Dr. Hensel, a generalist in the South, is "painfully aware of how many issues I am expected to address in 'routine' history taking and physical examination. A partial list includes screening for depression, alcohol abuse, tobacco abuse, incontinence, sexual dysfunction, physical or emotional abuse, and the desirability of advanced directives."

Every one of these pieces of information is no doubt important and has strong, vocal advocates. One attorney who is an expert and active in the field of sexual and spousal abuse has stated publicly that she is prepared to "take to court" any doctors who do not ask each patient about such abuse. Assuming that your primary-care doctor is well informed on each of these issues, are you or your health plan prepared to pay for the hour or more needed to explain all of these issues? Would you even want to discuss for an hour these topics, whether you are interested or not? The doctor in this regard feels that "you are damned if you do and damned if you don't." This raises several interesting points. If society decides that each doctor must spend much more time with the patient, we will have to train many more physicians, rather than the smaller number presently envisioned.

Every physician has the fear, made worse by the pressure of time, of missing some of the well-known deceivers of diagnosis, such as pulmonary embolism, obscure infectious diseases, addictions, hidden cancers, and incipient psychoses. Diagnosis is never one hundred percent certain. As Dr. Martin F. Sturman said in an April 1995 letter to the editors of the *Annals of Internal Medicine*, "Experienced clinicians have always known that diagnostic certainty is an idiot's chimera and the cause of untold mischief." Dr. Eric J. Cassell commented in the *New England Journal of Medicine*, in June 1995, "We want doctors to function as well when they are tired as when they are rested, to admit error freely to themselves and others, to care more about the patients being okay than about whether they are right. . . ." In other words, it is very hard to be a good doctor.

The doctor must balance a physician's polite and trusting acceptance of the patient's perception of an illness with the slightly adversarial attitude of a lawyer—that is to say to him- or herself, "What else could it be?" For example, a professor appeared at a university health clinic late on a busy Friday during the influenza season. The doctor asked, "What is wrong?" The patient said, "I feel terrible. I have the flu, I guess." This seemed logical at the time, and the doctor prescribed some cough medicine with codeine and bed rest. The patient went home and soon thereafter collapsed and died, presumably of a heart attack. To his family this was prima facie evidence of physician incompetence. It is not known whether the patient had premonitory symptoms such as chest pain, shortness of breath, palpitations, or a heavy sweat. The patient evidently did not volunteer that he was having such symptoms. In any case, the physician took the man at his word and did not ask detailed questions about other symptoms, nor did he do a cardiac examination.

All medical diagnosis rests on probability, never on certainty. Statistically speaking, the doctor's diagnosis of influenza would have been correct under the circumstances 95 percent of the time. In this case several adverse factors entered into the sad outcome. The patient did not volunteer much information. The physician did not persist in taking time to ask for more details. The patient did not insist on a more thorough examination. The expectation of very serious disease in a university clinic is very low. The vast majority of students and most of the faculty are quite healthy. In this case, the death could have been caused by a previously unanticipated coronary artery closure. Also sudden cardiac deaths sometimes occur among influenza patients during an epidemic. We will never know whether a more self-aware and insistent patient, meeting with an inquisitive and unhurried physician, would have resulted in a different outcome.

To err is human; for a practicing physician to err, no matter how infrequently, is inevitable. In this era of litigation, where every adverse happening is often blamed on someone else and monetary compensation is demanded, the threat of lawsuit hangs over every doctor and has added new layers of complexity and expense to practice. The cost of malpractice insurance ranges from $6,000 to over $100,000 a year—a cost passed on to the patients and their health-care plans.

Physicians are now educated in risk management, which has become part of most continuing-education requirements. In a recent series of lectures at the Harvard Medical Institution's Risk Management Foundation, typical topics, based on actual claims, included "Difficult Patients and Situations," "Surgery under Managed Care," "Obstetrical Mishaps," "Medication Errors," "Emergency Care," and "Confidentiality." The primary-care physician faces some unique dilemmas because of the threat of lawsuits. If he uses an answering machine, how often must he check it? If he prescribes over the telephone, especially when covering for another doctor, how can he be aware of the patient's ailments and idiosyncrasies? If the third-party insurer refuses payment for the patient, the doctor may in some cases be responsible for payment. Physicians who have been sued, even if they are completely exonerated, inevitably suffer anxiety and depression, and many leave medical practice forever. Suicides of physicians who have been the subject of a malpractice action are not rare.

In the long run, your best assurance in the selection of a doctor comes from friends who know the doctor personally, within the profession and outside. A new arrival in a large city cannot know this. The reputation of the doctor's hospital connections, the medical school he or she attended, and especially the hospitals where the doctor later trained, are a good but not an infallible guide.

Nurses

TRENDS IN NURSING

Even as the status and duties of physicians are changing rapidly, so are those of nurses. In some areas nurses are in demand as trained primary-care health providers, but on the whole there is widespread unemployment. In 1970 there were 750,000 R.N.'s, but by 1992 the number had risen to 1,853,000. The Pew Health Professions Commission predicted in 1995 that one in every five medical and nursing schools will be closed by the year 2000.

Within and outside of the nursing profession there is a debate over the duties and levels of responsibilities that should be assumed by nurses. Bills already passed by, or before, several state legislatures would permit qualified R.N.'s to have independent practice and prescribing privileges. Some think R.N.'s with additional specialized training can and should be permitted to do much of the work now done by physicians. Others feel that nurses should do more of the traditional daily care in hospitals, nursing homes, and patients' homes, working entirely under the direction of physicians.

The title R.N. (registered nurse) is not an academic degree but a certification of fitness to practice issued by a state board of nursing after the candidate can present suitable credentials and pass an examination. An L.P.N. (licensed practical nurse) must have a high-school diploma and be a graduate from an approved program, usually of two years' duration. For specialized nurses the requirements for training, licensure as an R.N., and continuing education in most places require more money and a bigger investment of time than ever. R.N.'s with this background quite understandably feel that they deserve more pay, higher status, job security, and permission to function independently.

There are a number of specialized nursing positions requiring extra schooling and training. To become a nurse practitioner, a student must earn an R.N. degree, a bachelor's degree, and an M.A. or an M.S. in nursing, and in over half of the states, certification is required by the American Nursing Association. A certified nurse-midwife (C.N.M.), needs a further one and a half to two years of specialized education after the R.N. degree, in a certified program. Certified nurse anesthetists (C.N.A.) must follow their R.N. degree by two or three years of additional training and then national board

examinations. Compared to the R.N.'s who have only the basic certification, these nurse specialists have better chances of employment
at present, with more benefits and better salaries. In most states, certified nurse practitioners, nurse midwives, and nurse anesthetists
are entitled to bill separately for their services and receive third-
party (such as Blue Shield) payments.

With many health-care issues still unresolved, the managed-care,
profit-and-loss orientation of the medical field has thrown nursing
into turmoil. An article by Ellen D. Baer, R.N., in the *American
Journal of Nursing* carries the headline MONEY MANAGERS ARE UN-
RAVELING THE TAPESTRY OF NURSING. Hospitals, faced with shorter
inpatient stays and more empty beds, have laid off nurses by the
thousands. In many cases, experienced and highly trained nurses
have been replaced by lower-paid, less-qualified workers. Licensed
practical nurses do much of the work formerly done by R.N.'s.
Aides with little or no training or education, in turn, do much of
the work formerly done by L.P.N.'s, just short of administering
medications, giving injections, and charting patients' health data.
Usually those nurses who have kept their jobs in hospitals are asked
to cover more patients during each shift. The strain on the nurses
is great, and the possibility of error due to haste is increased. The
patient gets less hands-on caring attention. It should not be a surprise, then, to find that hospital nurses and aides feel unhappy and
that patients often feel neglected.

HEALTH CARE SETTINGS FOR NURSES

Another special area of nursing is home care. To provide for trained
nursing in a patient's home, with nurses sometimes working in
shifts to cover twenty-four hours a day, is beyond the pocketbooks
of almost any American, and very few people have insurance that
covers such services. Home health care is increasingly best man-

aged by firms that are "vertically integrated," that is, by an administrative office that employs consulting doctors, R.N.'s, L.P.N.'s, laboratory technicians, intravenous nurse specialists, nurse clinical specialists, and other specialists as needed. Terminal care and cancer chemotherapy, for example, can be well managed at home by such an arrangement. Many nurses enjoy this sort of home care work, but many more do not.

In convalescent homes and rehabilitation hospitals and homes, most of the supervisory work is done by registered nurses, with a greater or lesser degree of specialized training in various types of therapy. Here again, money is the stumbling block. Third party payors, notably Medicare and Medicaid, closely regulate the criteria for admission and payment to these institutions. By setting limits on reimbursement, the payors force the institution to economize on salaries. Lower-salaried workers replace R.N.'s wherever this is legally possible.

Nursing homes and the medical-care facilities attached to many retirement communities also employ nurses with various levels of training. Each state has its own regulations; many require that one fully trained and licensed R.N. be present for at least one shift every day. Once again, the bottom-line financial consideration is paramount in the facility's choice of caregivers. The more care given by lower-paid helpers, the fewer trained nurses have to be hired. This can result in heavy responsibility as well as hard work for the R.N. in charge.

These same observations apply to nurses working in schools and colleges and to the many thousands of nurses working in our jails and prisons. Nursing in jails and prisons attracts a large number of highly competent workers, who enjoy considerable autonomy. In many jails, juvenile detention centers, and prisons, the initial examinations, health-care appraisals, and daily sick line are in the hands of nurse practitioners. Over a thousand correctional nurses attend at least one of the national conferences on correctional health care each year. Many have passed the examinations for the coveted title of Certified Correctional Health Care Professional.

I have seen many nurses who enjoy institutional work. They do it conscientiously and keep up their skills by continuing education. Other nurses are not able to deal every day with dependent, incontinent, complaining, sometimes demented, sometimes hostile, elderly people or rebellious or disrespectful young people. Nurses contemplating this kind of work need to look into each correctional institution or nursing home as carefully as should families considering placement of their loved ones.

Added Risks in Nursing

A relatively recent hazard has been added to the difficulties of the nursing profession—the threat of malpractice. The Nurses Professional Liability Program lists seven "legal pitfalls," which include responsibility for:

1. Observing symptoms and reactions of patients, and taking prompt action when indicated.
2. Properly using all equipment.
3. Accurately recording all patient-care matters, such as dosages, times, readings, etc. Human error is not an acceptable defense.
4. Supervising others under them who are engaged in nursing care. Nurses can be sued for other nurses' mistakes.
5. Carrying out "proper nursing procedure." (But what is "proper"?) Nurses can be sued either for following orders, or for using their own judgment.
6. Patient teaching and instruction.
7. Carrying out the orders of doctors—and for understanding the reason for, and the effect of, such orders. A doctor's mistake could find the nurse sharing the blame.

Since there is no limitation on the number of people named in a malpractice suit, nurses are often included along with the doctors and the hospital.

In short, nursing is potentially rewarding, but it can be hard to be a nurse. The future role of nursing in our health-care system is not at all clear.

Other Health Professionals

PHYSICIAN ASSISTANTS (P.A.'S)

There are now 25,000 P.A.'s, licensed in all fifty states. Their training requires two years of college, followed in most cases by a two-year course divided between didactic teaching and supervised practice. P.A.'s work in doctors' offices carrying out orders, assisting with procedures, preparing medications, taking histories, and keeping up the medical records, all this under the direct supervision of the doctors. In rural practices, P.A.'s often make house calls and assess the need for further care. Many go on to further training to become emergency technicians or R.N.'s. Other P.A.'s are happy to continue working at the lower level, enjoying the patient contact and rapport with the physicians. With a competent P.A., a physician can often take better care of a larger number of patients.

PHYSICAL THERAPISTS

These professionals typically have five or six years of training after high school, four years of college, and a master's degree. They work under supervision in hospitals or on physicians' orders in other organizations. In a large hospital physical therapy is a separate department, often headed by a physiatrist, who is a physician trained and certified in rehabilitation medicine.

OCCUPATIONAL THERAPISTS

In large teaching hospitals or rehabilitation clinics, both nonprofit and for-profit, occupational therapists do work that may overlap considerably with that of physical therapists. Their mandate originally was to help those people disabled at birth or by illness or injury to master skills enabling them to be employable and to be able to live by themselves. Most insurance plans and managed-care organizations do not permit occupational therapists to work as private practitioners, but only under doctors' orders and usually on a salary.

SPORTS MEDICINE PRACTITIONERS

Sports medicine is also a field that is increasingly popular for patients, doctors, and therapists. Many sports medicine clinics or physicians, usually orthopedic surgeons, employ therapists extensively, trained to a greater or lesser degree, very often by the physicians themselves. They are mostly physical or occupational therapists. The objects of sports medicine clinics are general conditioning, corrective and strengthening exercises, massage, heat, and other specialized techniques for the treatment of injuries. Increasingly, sports medicine aims at prevention of injury as well as treatment. This may involve the redesign of equipment and the teaching of new techniques of stretching and warming up, as well as preventive taping and bandaging. Under managed care, patient visits to sports medicine clinics will not be reimbursed unless the patient is referred by a primary-care doctor for treatment of a specific injury. The American College of Sports Medicine and the American Orthopedic Society for Sports Medicine have set up practice treatment guidelines for many injuries and other limiting conditions, and you can be sure that these will become more codified for the purposes of reimbursement by means of protocols that will specify the number and type of treatments.

Some physical therapists and occupational therapists work independently, and their patients pay them directly without necessarily expecting reimbursement. Such therapists must be licensed by the state. In some communities such therapists are required to register, be licensed, and to maintain their own equipment and place of work subject to inspection. It is well for you to find out from your town or city hall whether or not a therapist whom you are considering seeing is listed on their rolls and what qualifications he or she possesses. Of course, if your health plan pays for physical therapy ordered by a physician, be sure to follow the plan's rules.

EMERGENCY MEDICAL TECHNICIANS (E.M.T.'s)

E.M.T.'s, so often seen in television dramas, must have a high-school diploma and pass a state certification examination, after at least one semester of classes, lectures, and demonstrations, as well as at least ten hours of supervised hospital observation.

SPEECH THERAPISTS

Another form of professional caregiver is the speech therapist. Speech therapy is really a branch of neurological treatment and requires extensive training. The principal patients are people who are disabled by strokes, brain injury, or the removal of the vocal cords because of cancer, or disabled by congenital malformation of the mouth and throat. Speech therapists usually work in a nonprofit or for-profit organization, and under most health plans, patients seeking reimbursement can only see a speech therapist by referral either from the primary-care physician or some other appropriate specialist physician.

Treatment for learning disabilities is even more closely tied up with neurological training of a greater or lesser degree. In some states the law requires that the school system supply and pay for specially trained experts for students with various developmental delays. Learning disabilities, notably dyslexia, require a long period of treatment, and the results are often disappointingly slow and discouraging. Treatment in groups led by therapists who are usually trained at the master's or doctoral level is widespread and often quite successful. In some areas third-party insurance or managed care will pay for some of the treatment of learning disabilities, but since the treatment and training must extend over a period of years, sometimes a lifetime, it is expensive regardless of who pays for it.

NON-M.D. PSYCHOLOGICAL TREATMENT

There is no agreement as to who should treat people with psychotic, emotional, or neurotic ailments. There are, in addition to psychiatrists (M.D.'s), psychiatric social workers and clinical psychologists with various degrees of training and experience. In today's medical economic climate psychiatrists are facing a shrinking number of referral visits and lowered payments. Sometimes they feel that they must make a choice between practicing pharmacotherapy, such as prescribing antidepressants and tranquilizers, and the traditional analytically oriented "talk" therapy. Most psychiatrists now in practice try to do a little of both. Patients are often in a quandary as to whom to select, if indeed they have any choice.

Increasingly in managed-care organizations the referral will come from either a primary-care doctor or a salaried official of the managed-care organization, usually a mental-health specialist who does not do treatment, but who decides which people need psychological help and how many sessions will be allowed and paid for.

The person making this decision rarely meets the patient in person and sometimes never even speaks to him or her on the telephone. Psychotherapists who have not earned the M.D. degree have the disadvantage of not being trained to identify organic disease. People with AIDS, multiple sclerosis, or brain tumors, for example, may appear to suffer from behavior disorders, and the delay in receiving proper treatment during a period of psychotherapy can be harmful, as well as a waste of money.

Clinical Psychologists

A clinical psychologist is a therapist who generally has received a master's or doctoral degree from a college or university and has received further clinical training. Managed-care plans use many such mental-health professionals because they are paid less than a physician psychiatrist. Clinical psychologists are particularly helpful in testing people for diagnostic purposes at both ends of the age spectrum: children and the aged. Children may need testing for intellectual and/or emotional impairment, and old people for determining the presence of dementias such as Alzheimer's. The mentally retarded and learning disabled are also tested by these professionals to determine their strengths and weaknesses.

Clinical psychologists who are independent caregivers often advertise their practices in newspapers and magazines for the general public; physician psychiatrists still very seldom do direct advertising. Licensed to practice psychotherapy in most states, clinical psychologists are not permitted, however, to prescribe medication. In managed care, many times the primary-care doctor, rather than a trained psychiatrist, is, therefore, often asked to prescribe powerful antidepressants, tranquilizers, or antipsychotic medicines as needed for a patient whom he or she hardly knows, because it has been requested by the psychologist. The responsibility and the liability thus incurred is one more stress for the family doctor.

Psychiatric Nurse Clinicians

In addition to the R.N., psychiatric nurse clinicians have a bachelor's degree and a master's degree in psychiatric nursing. They can treat patients directly and receive third-party payments.

Psychiatric Social Workers and Licensed Independent Clinical Social Workers

These mental-health professionals have, in general, a master's degree, beyond the bachelor's, and in many states they are permitted to practice diagnosis and psychotherapy under separate licensing arrangements, without referral from an M.D. Schools of social work provide clinical training in addition to academic work. As a patient, you should find out in advance the licensure status of a prospective psychiatric social worker, his or her level of training, and preferably any membership in professional associations or certification before deciding to undergo treatment with that person. It should go without saying that you should find out whether your health plan will pay for such treatment, and if so, for how many visits.

For emotional or mental-health problems under managed-care plans, the patient may indeed have very little choice, so it is difficult to make a general recommendation as to what sort of therapist you should seek. An examination by a physician should be a first step, to exclude the possibility of organic disease as the cause of symptoms. Again, if you have a good relationship with an experienced primary-care physician, you may be guided. In managed-care organizations that have an entirely separate mental-health referral system, the primary-care physician may not have any input. People vary so greatly, and their problems are so different, that finding the "right" therapist is often a matter of chance. The best referral would come from an experienced generalist or family doctor who knows both you and the system. Friends who have been under treatment may have some useful thoughts, but they may also have biases that may not be helpful. The clergy, at present, have usually had some pastoral training in clinical settings, and experience in their daily pastoral work may enable them to suggest names of therapists.

The large public and private mental hospitals for long-term treatment are primarily for people with major mental illnesses such as severe degrees of the bipolar (manic-depressive) condition or schizophrenia. Other institutions specialize in problems of addiction, usually to alcohol, but also to heroin, cocaine, and other substances. Most large state mental-health hospitals are staffed by a mix of M.D.'s, psychologists, and psychiatric social workers. In the 1960s and 1970s a great wave of deinstitutionalization put many helpless people inadequately equipped to cope with life into communities and on to the streets, where they are unable to care for themselves, and communities are unable to care for them. Many are now the homeless, and, sad to say, many are in prison.

Obviously, finding the proper avenues to help people with emotional and mental disturbances is confusing and difficult. It takes persistence and patience to understand the options available and sound advice wherever it can be found as to the plan to follow. The interests of these mental-health professionals and of the patients are the same, and it will require joint effort over a period of years to reverse the damaging downsizing of institutions and mental-health clinics that is now taking place.

NUTRITIONISTS

There are a relatively small number of physicians who have had special training in nutrition and who confine their practice to such diagnosis and treatment. A physician engaged in the practice of nutrition needs a very large referral base, and before consulting one the patient should find out the cost and mechanism for payment. Most nutritionists, however, are not physicians. Schools of nutrition exist in many universities and teaching hospitals. Becoming a nutritionist requires one, two, or even three years of training beyond the bachelor's degree, and such nutritionists work largely for hospitals or clinics on a salary arrangement. They see patients only on referral. Some of the bewildering varieties of therapists and systems for dealing with life's many problems caused by eating will appear in chapter 8.

ETHICISTS

Until recently, the only people who were principally concerned with medical ethics full-time were academic philosophers and clergy. Now many medical schools and hospitals have staff members, full- or part-time, whose function is to make judgments on ethical issues and to help physicians and students to understand the issues.

Ethicists are heavily involved in medical-school teaching. Some are doctors of medicine who have received special training in institutions such as the Hastings Institute in New York. Many divinity schools and other theological teaching institutions have become active participants in medical decision making. Some issues ethicists address would include the right to die, the right to refuse treatment, decision making in regard to abortion, the use of experimental treatments, and radical and unconventional treatment of emotional or behavioral disorders. Ethicists are not employed directly by the patient, but they are often involved, and in some instances by law, in helping families make such difficult decisions. Patients and their families who need to make hard decisions or face other difficult dilemmas should inquire as to the availability of such trained people who are often members of an established, multidisciplinary hospital committee.

Exercise Guidance

Up to this point, we have been discussing health-care professionals, working within the conventional and established systems. Since good health is everyone's concern, the line between amateurs and professionals can become blurred. If health-care professionals deal largely with the deviations from the normal, sickness of one sort or another, they are not the sole custodians of good health. Exercise, fitness training, and all the apparatus (and costumes) involved with them constitute a major industry in this country, and exercise is almost a national mania. Health clubs are available in almost every community; their objective is "well-being." Whether this means to the subscriber a better self-image, large muscles, greater endurance, a deep tan, enhanced sexual powers, or merely recreation and companionship is a matter of choice. The local chapter of the American College of Sports Medicine may make recommendations for those desiring a greater degree of fitness, under defined and standardized conditions.

4

Health Care: How It Is Delivered

Our little systems have their day.

ALFRED, LORD TENNYSON, *In Memoriam*

Health care constitutes one of America's largest financial involvements: Americans spent $942 billion on health care in 1993; the industry employs 10 million people, among whom are 2 million nurses, 650,000 doctors, and 150,000 dentists. There were 126 medical schools, 6,600 hospitals, and 25,600 nursing-care facilities in 1993, according to the U.S. Department of Commerce. In other words, this is a gigantic enterprise, and these figures do not even take into account the millions of people and the 13 billion dollars involved in the delivery of unconventional or alternative care.

The large sums have inevitably attracted investment capital. Privatization of all aspects of health care is growing at an ever faster rate. The federal, state, and local governments have their own fiscal concerns and increasingly "privatize" formerly state-supported services. The appeal of this trend rests on the popular assumption that private industry can deliver services of quality comparable to or better than those offered by a city, county, state, or national government. Proponents and opponents of privatization both claim to have the best statistics, but their figures do not, to my mind, give a clear answer. To sell a money-losing tax-supported city, county, or federal hospital to a corporation that will pay taxes while at the same time promising to maintain an undiminished, high quality of care sounds too good to be true. Common sense suggests that services will be cut, especially to those who most need help. All of us must keep a close and skeptical eye on these changes. Although I concede that government agencies may be overstaffed and inefficient in some cases, I believe that within five years public outrage will bring about restoration of tax support for health care under government supervision.

In addition to the federal and state governments' involvement in this huge enterprise, there are, according to the Department of Commerce, approximately 1,100 health-insurance companies. Space and time do not allow description of the benefits offered by these 1,100 plans. By next year they will probably mostly be changed by mergers and acquisitions. We now spend 14 percent of our gross domestic product on health care, up from 6 percent in 1965. To people who pay all their own health-insurance premiums as well as other medical and dental bills not covered by their policy, these are not just statistics; they are terrifying realities. In 1993 total health expenditures were $3,300 per person, and over $13,000 a year for a family of four, and it is by far the highest health-care expenditure in the world.

In any other business, the customer knows in advance the price, quality, and quantity of a product he or she is getting, but not so in health care. The prices paid for services are largely determined by third-party providers, both private and public (such as Medicare and Medicaid). There are fewer and fewer individual private practitioners who are paid cash for each procedure (fee for service). For everyone else third-party providers aim at cutting costs by limiting the fees paid and the services provided.

People looking for a doctor in America today have to choose one from the particular health plan they or their employer have selected. Americans receive health care from a variety of different sources, financed by many different mechanisms. The details are often confusing or poorly explained if at all, but it is important to understand the basic differences. Health care is provided by public, private, for-profit, and nonprofit institutions, including hospitals, individual doctors' offices, clinics, nursing homes, and specialized facilities such as those for alcoholism, mental illness, and tuberculosis. The financing is as varied as are the places where people receive care. Traditionally the patient paid cash out of pocket, or received a bill, for each service. Over the past fifty years this form of "fee-for-service" arrangement has been supplemented by an insurance payment for each service, the money coming either from a nonprofit corporation, such as Blue Cross and Blue Shield, or from a commercial insurer. Over the past fifty years, and especially within the last five years, more and more people have received medical care as members or subscribers to some form of managed care.

Access

Health services are of no value if patients have no access to them, whether the cause be limited hours, lack of walk-in facilities, or difficulty in transportation. Refusal of the service plan to authorize any out-of-town treatment, or to pay for use of emergency services in another nearby location without extensive negotiation also limits the availability of the care which has been prepaid. Requiring a co-payment also effectively limits access to health care for poor people. In 1975 Romer and colleagues demonstrated that reduction in this so-called ambulatory access led to higher hospitalization rates. The Rand Health Insurance Experiment reported in the *New England Journal of Medicine* in 1986 that reductions in accessibility to medical care had various harmful effects on people's health. People who do not have a primary-care physician likewise get less care and in the end have more expensive illnesses.

People who have little money and no insurance tend to go, if at all, only to emergency rooms, which are very expensive organizations and are not designed in any way to give routine, unhurried care. In many states physicians and hospitals may not refuse care to anyone regardless of the person's ability to pay. So, in theory at least, every American can receive care, but various obstacles can often prevent this. Some physicians and clinics simply refuse to see people who are not insured unless they pay cash up front. Many primary-care providers refuse to take Medicaid patients because of the low and slow payments. However, in some states, refusal to accept Medicaid patients may lead to revocation of the doctor's license to practice.

The Medicaid Access Study Group in 1994 called to make appointments for patients with one of three common conditions, namely, back pain, dysuria (painful urination), and sore throat. They sampled 953 practice sites, and in over 44 percent of these settings patients on Medicaid were not given an appointment. When these same sites were called six weeks later, the caller posing as a privately insured patient, 60 percent got appointments within two days. Urgent-care centers and clinics gave more appointments to Medicaid patients than did private practices. Forty percent of the sites called demanded a mandatory copayment ranging from $1 to $200. The group reported, however, that in some cases financial hardship was recognized and the fee was waived.

I have had several patients who have lost their health insurance and could not buy any coverage because of joblessness or pre-existing disease. This is not the way Americans should treat each other. We urgently need national legislation and probably subsidation to cover those in a high-risk pool.

What Is Managed Care?

Before we look at the settings where you can receive health-care services, an overview of managed care is in order. The key phrase in all discussions of health in this country at present and in the foreseeable future is "managed care." This system covers many different types of plans. All plans have in common prepayment for comprehensive health care of all sorts. According to the American Society of Internal Medicine, managed care has the following features: A network of contractors provides health-care services. Patients are directed to contracted health-care providers, and their benefits are limited or not valid if they use noncontract providers, that is, if they visit a doctor outside their health-care plan, they have to pay out of pocket. Utilization management and quality assurance systems are in place. The financial risk is shared by both patients and health-care providers. The most prevalent form of managed care is the HMO, or health maintenance organization, which will be discussed later in this chapter. It is a form of managed care in which everyone must choose a primary-care physician who has signed a contract with that specific HMO and who must give approval for any referrals to specialists.

Attempts have been made to define "primary care" since the British National Health Service did so seventy years ago, defining it as "the essential, continuous care necessary for general well-being and the care of common problems provided in a community setting." This definition was made the centerpiece by the World Health Organization in 1978 in their recommendations on health care. The primary-care doctor essentially bears the responsibility for organizing and directing patient care. The Institute of Medicine, which is a division of the independent National Academy of Sciences in this country, in 1978 defined the duties of the primary-care doctor: being the patient's first contact with the medical system, offering comprehensive services, assuming continuous responsibility, coordinating the care, and assuming accountability.

Health-Care Delivery Systems

Once you have enrolled in a plan and reviewed the rules and regulations, you can then study your options for seeking health-care services, based on what settings you prefer, keeping in mind that all services must be cleared through your plan. Following is a brief description of the various means of receiving health care.

PRIVATE DOCTORS

Private, self-employed physicians are paid either directly by the patient or by billing the insurer (under a so-called indemnity plan). The doctor bills the insurance company and is paid (indemnified) by it. This is the traditional pattern, being gradually replaced by various managed-care arrangements. Independent doctors are not reimbursed through managed care. Fifty or sixty years ago, when 95 percent of American doctors were general practitioners and mostly male, practicing usually alone but sometimes with one or two partners, the relationship between patient and doctor was clear and the process straightforward. Market forces played a role in private practice. You picked a doctor, and if you liked him you stuck with him. The doctor's ability to acquire and retain patients depended to a large extent on mutual satisfaction, which often led to friendship and mutual trust.

The doctor kept long hours and worked six or seven days a week. There was no requirement for continuing education and no ongoing surveillance of the doctor's competence. The office was often chaotic. State regulations were few, so records were often incomplete, the laboratory unsupervised, and the referral system haphazard. The doctor had free choice of referrals to specialists, often using friends because they were nearby, accessible, and cooperative. If the patient went to the hospital, his G.P. was in charge. Full, unlimited admitting privileges were extended to all doctors who were on staff at the hospital. If the case was too complex for the doctor, he could call on his favorite specialist or transfer the patient to a larger hospital with more specialized facilities. The indications for consulting, admission, and transfer were largely unregulated. There were few limitations on the scope of the doctor's activities; a state license authorized then, and still does, a physician to do any operation or order any treatment he wished. Few institutions outside of the teaching hospitals maintained rigorous internal controls on supervision. No one inspected the doctor's records, or his office.

All of this has changed, and in terms of quality of care, for the better. The private physician who depends on fee-for-service income (with the exception of a few well-known specialists) faces a smaller practice and less income. Most of his potential patients are rapidly becoming covered under a managed-care or insurance plan, and cannot get reimbursed for seeing him if he is not in the plan. As a result, doctors both young and old, but especially the young, are working for managed-care organizations, gaining in security what they have lost in autonomy. Older physicians are either continuing on but with a smaller income and practice, or else retiring early.

Since managed care has brought with it training, supervision, and surveillance of doctors, thereby creating a better quality of health care and a weeding out of the incompetent, everyone should be happy, but that is not the case. Patients have less choices, and so do physicians.

PREFERRED PROVIDER ORGANIZATIONS

There are private, self-employed groups of physicians whose situation is similar to that of the solo practitioners except that the group may incorporate. In some cases the doctors share fees and negotiate with the hospital or insurance plan as a preferred provider organization (PPO), receiving referrals from the plan in return for using that hospital or plan's specialty network and services. There are many variations of this type of organization. One advantage to the doctors is that they can be covered if they need to take time off. This means that the patient may not always see his or her own doctor, but continuity of care and exchange of information are obviously more easily managed in a small group than in a solo practice. The doctors in a PPO are members usually of Blue Shield and other health-insurance plans. These group practices are at present being bought out, particularly in California and the Northeast, by large integrated managed-care plans, and the group's doctors now work for a plan, which offers some degree of job security.

At a three-day meeting in Boston, Massachusetts, in September 1995, the topic of which was "Primary-Care Medicine in the Age of Managed Care," one doctor in attendance asked the director of a large health plan why a group of physicians could not set up and operate their own plan, so that they could practice the way they thought best. The reply, from Dr. David Nash, was that payors would not tolerate a plan that was not proven to be cost efficient. The criterion, he went on to say, of the investor-managers of health plans is, what works? This is probably true, yet some groups of doctors still hope to be able to set up plans that they can completely control.

INDEPENDENT PRACTICE ASSOCIATIONS

Independent practice associations (IPAs) are dwindling groups consisting of solo practitioners working under fee-for-service who band together in order to negotiate better terms with insurers and hospitals. Unfortunately doctors have not been trained to be experts in fiscal management or in the intricacies of mergers and acquisitions. Their ability to organize and to drive a bargain cannot match the experience of the financial managers of the for-profit managed care organizations. The for-profit concerns are free to set the financial terms of an agreement, but attempts by physicians to set fees have been considered to be in conflict with federal laws regarding price-fixing and restraint of trade. I have been present at many discussions where groups of practicing doctors have listened to experts explaining what they can and cannot do to organize to their advantage and to live within the constraints now existing. The discussions usually develop an adversarial tone, with the physicians reacting to their loss of independence and their sense that they can no longer practice medicine in a way that they consider to be in the best interest of their patients. I believe that these losses are at the root of the anger and unhappiness of many doctors, far more than any consideration of lower incomes. To look at health-care reform as being primarily an attempt to save money by giving less money to doctors is a dangerous oversimplification.

HEALTH MAINTENANCE ORGANIZATIONS

Health maintenance organizations (HMOs) are the fastest-growing type of health-care delivery system at present. Over forty million Americans are already covered by them. In return for a fixed sum paid in varying degrees by the individual, family, or employer, all generally accepted medical expenses are covered. In some plans, the covered patient may go to one of the private physicians on the panel; the doctor is reimbursed by the HMO on a fixed fee schedule. More commonly, the doctor is on a salary. Procedures or tests that are considered experimental or of unproven value are not paid for. As a result there are sometimes arguments and often lawsuits or legislative mandates (as in the question of whether to permit more than one day of hospitalization for routine obstetrical delivery).

The physicians in an HMO are usually paid a fixed salary with bonuses or penalties based on "productivity" after annual review. They are rewarded for giving fewer specialty referrals and ordering less expensive tests. In some HMOs physicians are paid, as in Great Britain, by "capitation"—that is, each doctor is paid a fixed fee monthly for each patient on his or her panel. The U.S. industry standard for a general physician's panel is 1,700 patients per doctor. Investors and plan managers like the capitation system because the income and expenses are more predictable, so capitation is becoming insurers' favored mechanism. You should try to find out how many other patients are on your doctor's panel by asking the sales representative of your plan.

The ratio of physicians to patients in an HMO may give an indication of doctor availability. HMOs in general have only about half as many doctors per thousand patients as are available in the general population. This economy of the system comes about in part by the greater use of nurse practitioners and general internists combined with sharply restricted referrals to specialists. Also, in part, this apparent saving results from exclusion of high-risk patients by various stratagems, such as refusing to accept patients with serious preexisting diseases or refusing to retain subscribers whose employment has ended.

The satisfaction of patients with 21 different health plans was studied in 1994 by the National Commission for Quality Assurance (NAQA). Eighty-four percent of the patients polled reported that they were satisfied. As reported in the *New York Times* of February 24, 1995, the "highest satisfaction"—96.8 percent—was achieved by the Blue Cross/Blue Shield Plan of Rochester, New York. Plans in Colorado, St. Louis, Pennsylvania, and Minneapolis were not far behind. The lowest rate of satisfaction reported by patients was with the Health Insurance Plan of Greater New York—72 percent, still an impressive number of favorable responses. These figures are hard to reconcile with the almost-universal dissatisfaction with the high cost of health care. As in many surveys, the manner in which the questions are asked can have a significant impact on the response. If the question were phrased, "If you should have to pay for the entire cost of your health care, would you still be satisfied?" the reported satisfaction might be quite different.

The "Freedom Plan"

Another type of plan of which the Oxford Plan, based in Norwalk, Connecticut, is among the first and most successful, blends managed care with freedom of choice of doctor. Its enrollment, according to the *New York Times,* doubled in the years 1994 and 1995 to a total of 1.16 million members. In this "Freedom Plan" the member can choose a doctor who is in the network, paying only a minimal fee for each visit, or the member can pay a deductible and pay a portion of the additional medical charges if he or she goes to any doctor he or she chooses. The premium as of April 1996 was 15 percent higher than that of the "pure" HMOs. Financial analysts are concerned that this plan's cash reserves may be insufficient to cover increased costs. As legislators hear the cries of those who cannot buy health insurance because of preexisting illness, age, or other adverse factors, it is likely that all plans may be compelled to accept higher-risk patients. This will, of course, drain the cash reserves and necessitate higher premiums for such plans.

Benefits to Patients under HMOs

Many studies have shown that in the HMO form of managed care, patients receive a high standard of care as measured, for example, by rates of children's immunizations, women's mammograms, and Pap smears. This shows enlightened self-interest, since testing can detect conditions that are more costly if treated later. Under managed care the performance of the doctors is routinely monitored, and the expenses resulting from the doctors' orders and referrals receive close scrutiny.

What can patients expect from physicians under managed care? Every HMO tries to have on its staff physicians who are well-trained, possessing excellent references, and possessing good personal qualifications. Most HMOs keep a statistical profile of each doctor, often a highly sophisticated analysis of time spent, costs of tests, number of referrals, number of patients hospitalized, errors in judgment, omission of essentials, and patient complaints. Although this surveillance makes some physicians feel uncomfortable and excessively regimented, the patient may expect benefits from certain measurements of quality. An incidental benefit is the demonstrated decrease in allegations of malpractice.

Managed care can help doctors practice better medicine. The HMO physician does not have to arrange coverage for his or her time off, and ongoing medical education is supported. Staff conferences and sharing of data can give the staff moral as well as professional support and a sense of solidarity. Indeed, the power of a united and organized staff is perhaps the best safeguard against excessive restraints on the practice of medicine by the money managers.

The layman can more easily judge the quality of care in a managed-care organization, because of its size and fiscal expertise, than the quality of care given by a solo practitioner. A potential female subscriber can (or should be able to) inquire about the percentage of women receiving Pap smears, mammograms, and the percentages of cesarean sections performed as well as the length of postpartum hospital stay allowed. Parents can be assured about the adequacy of routine checkups, completeness of immunizations, and the availability of specialist referrals for their children. Almost all managed-care organizations have a very good record, far better than our national average, when it comes to completeness of immunizations of the children of plan subscribers. Parents like to be able always to see the same pediatrician, but this is not always possible.

Challenges of HMOs

As more and more HMOs are owned by investors, the care of the patient as a human being may suffer. As Professor Adam Yarmolinsky has pointed out, "Physicians have a professional and indeed a moral commitment to the care of patients, . . . but when, as is increasingly the case, HMOs are established or purchased by insurance companies or other investor-owned businesses, physicians themselves become subject to the direction and control of entities that have not taken the Hippocratic Oath and for which the price of the stock and earnings per share may be more important than the welfare of patients."

For the physician practicing under a managed-care contract, there is a serious conflict: He or she is responsible by the nature of the doctor-patient relationship for the interests of the patient, acting as a fiduciary. Under the law, a fiduciary is held to the highest standards of conduct. But the managed-care plan at every level exerts pressure on the physician to keep costs down, by minimizing testing, specialists' consultation, and hospitalization. The doctor who accepts too many patients under a capitation plan may have to cut corners and skimp on patient time, but, on the other hand, limiting the size of one's panel can lead to an unacceptably small net income. Physician-owned HMOs may be in violation of the antitrust laws that aim at avoidance of price-fixing. Hospitals that own one HMO or more may also be at risk of losing their tax-exempt charitable status; here the for-profit firms have a substantial advantage.

Another potential conflict may arise when the doctor who is

legally and morally required to provide "informed consent" to his patient, fails to reveal the HMO's restrictions of service. For example, a physician may unwittingly fail to tell the patient all of the plan's restrictions on length of stay for various hospital procedures, such as normal delivery or hernia repair. The patient might then sue the doctor, saying that if he had been so informed, he would not have bought the plan. Physicians disclosing information that might cause patient dissatisfaction with the managed-care plan have been, in some cases, severely disciplined and even dismissed from the plan. This practice has been called a "gag rule," and it is a part of the contract signed by the doctor upon joining some plans. Some physicians disciplined in this manner have sued their plan. Legislation has been proposed to protect managed-care doctors who feel the obligation to inform their patients of deficiencies in coverage.

The Future of HMOs

As HMOs compete more and more to become attractive to everyone, the public may ask for and expect some improvements. For example, patients want physicians and nurses whose ethnic background, language, and culture is similar to theirs. Such caregivers are at present in considerable demand by managed-care organizations. Medical Spanish is taught in some medical schools and sponsored by at least one HMO, as translators are in short supply in most managed-care operations.

As competition and public exposure increase, we can look for more cooperation and consideration from the HMO staffs. Access to care will, or should, become simpler and quicker. The quality of care, if measured by the preventive measures mentioned above, will undoubtedly continue to be high. The quality of care, if measured by easy access to the doctor or sympathetic listening may be something else. Professor Leonard Laster, writing in the *Boston Globe*, reminds us that "as the universal panacea the legislators have embraced managed care. Every so often, one of them remembers to as-sure us that their brave new programs will certainly preserve the quality of our care. Hogwash . . . let the patient beware."

Managed-care plans, which will eventually enroll most Americans, may well result in better health. The reason for this is that intense research into costs of illness in recent years has clearly demon-strated that better health for all brings about a lower cost to society. For example, some excellent cooperative studies in Minnesota have demonstrated that the cost to the health plan, by month or by year, of smokers is double that of nonsmokers. Obesity also is correlated with twice the health-care costs of normal weight. Profit-minded investors can see the logic of lowering the incidence of the resulting diabetes, lung cancer, and heart disease. The challenge to everyone is in finding ways to reduce obesity and smoking. Many managed-care plans are already actively encouraging prevention and early intervention by educating their physicians and nurses in making compliance a part of their physicians' evaluations.

HOSPITAL-BASED PRACTICES

Hospital-controlled and hospital-based practices are also prevalent. They are financed both by indemnity insurance (fee for service) and by arrangements with health insurance or managed-care orga-nizations. Here available special services are restricted to those per-formed by the hospital's staff. In a small hospital this may be a major disadvantage, but in a large institution, such as the Mayo Clinic or most of our nation's large teaching hospitals, every service of the best quality is on hand. This arrangement can work well if the patient's primary-care provider (doctor or nurse) is available to provide continuity as well as a caring, personal touch. A case man-ager who can track the patient's course through various specialty clinics is invaluable; we hope that the case-manager system will be more widely adopted. Some managed-care plans find that case managers have effectively saved money by facilitating procedures and consultations.

PUBLIC CLINICS

Public clinics in the inner city are generally funded by Medicaid with contributions from the city and the state. Their patients seldom have health insurance. There is usually a stated fee, which is sometimes paid in part, but usually not. The staff is usually devoted, underpaid, overworked, and far more competent than more affluent suburbanites might think. Some of the finest nurses, doctors, and social workers of my acquaintance work in such clinics. It is here that the day-to-day struggles against contagious disease, the effects of substance abuse, underage pregnancy, homelessness, malnutrition, and interpersonal violence are dealt with. Here there is no line dividing physical and mental illness from the effects of poverty, broken family, and chronic unemployment. The administrators, doctors, and nurses have common goals; prestige and high incomes are not a factor. Understandably burnout is a problem; the less-hardy nurses and doctors drop out after a time.

Those medical and nursing students who have been assigned to rotations in these inner-city clinics (and sometimes in prisons and state mental hospitals) have a broadened view of the total needs of the population. The people who attend these clinics—the patients—think they have no alternatives. They are often ignorant of the ways in which they can take care of themselves and of the ways they might best use the health-care delivery system. Their assigned social workers usually face an excessively heavy case load, so it should come as no surprise when it is revealed that serious needs are unmet, and that some unfortunate people suffer needlessly because they do not understand the system and do not know how to get what they need. Many studies have demonstrated that underfunding these clinics results in the long run in expensive hospitalization, medications, even surgery to repair the effects of earlier neglect.

WALK-IN CENTERS

Freestanding, for-profit walk-in centers, sometimes known as "doc-in-a-box," have arisen largely in urban areas in response to the desire for round-the-clock accessibility with a minimum of waiting, in areas handy to public transportation or with easy parking. Such establishments may be owned by the individual practitioners, or by a local investor group, hospital, or HMO. The physicians are often "moonlighting" from positions in research or residency training. Characteristically these walk-in centers have advertising out front that emphasizes the fact that there is no need for making appointments and that there is a minimum amount of waiting.

The usual procedure is that on arriving you fill out a form and pay prior to being seen and treated. The fee may be reimbursed later by your health insurance, but usually it is not. As your HMO cannot control utilization, testing, and referrals at a walk-in center, the plan will not pay for voluntary use of the "doc-in-a-box." Patients are not likely to receive continuity of care or follow-up from such clinics. In short, a walk-in center may be just the thing you want for what appears to be a minor and immediate problem, but the buyer should be aware, and if possible do research into the walk-in center and find out about its general reputation in the community before visiting the clinic. Since such operations must be licensed as businesses and in most states as clinics, their ownership and other essential information should be on file either with the local or state Board of Health or medical institutional licensing facility.

MENTAL-HEALTH HOSPITALS

State hospitals for mental illness receive money from Medicare and Medicaid, private insurance, the state, and often the patients themselves. Admission is usually arranged through the mental-health system clinic or an individual psychiatrist. The downsizing of these hospitals beginning in the 1970s has brought about restricted admissions and earlier discharges, putting a correspondingly increased burden on mental-health clinics and individual therapists. The strong civil rights movement of the 1960s and 1970s made the involuntary commitment of psychotic men and women more difficult in most states, and voluntary commitment is now the rule (except in cases of criminal conviction).

For-profit mental hospitals have increasingly appealed to investors and major health-care corporations, as they now house many of those who were formerly in public institutions. Since private mental hospitals can choose whom to accept, they profit from securing paying patients. Over the years, past and present, many private mental hospitals have helped pay for the deficits of the large general hospitals that owned them. Some large nonprofit private mental hospitals are losing large amounts of money, however, on free care, although they are not obligated to accept patients who are on Medicare or Medicaid.

PUBLIC CHRONIC-CARE HOSPITALS

Public chronic-disease hospitals have traditionally cared for people with tuberculosis. Chemotherapy brought their census to an all-time low in 1993. Effective therapy in most cases not only greatly speeded recovery from tuberculosis, but rendered the patients non-contagious in a few weeks, so they could be safely released to their homes. In 1972 there were 72 tuberculosis hospitals, and by 1993 only 4. Now drug-resistant contagious tuberculosis is on the increase, and some long-closed units in hospitals will have to be reopened. The susceptibility of AIDS patients to tuberculosis has contributed substantially to the spread of that disease, especially drug-resistant strains. It is a challenge to treat both illnesses simultaneously, and these chronic-disease hospitals have been forced to acquire new expertise as have the practitioners on their staffs. Admission to such public chronic-disease hospitals is financed by a mix of public funds, health insurance, and managed-care contributions.

VETERANS ADMINISTRATION HEALTH CARE

The U.S. Veterans Administration operates a very large health-care system. It was originally intended for veterans with service-connected disabilities, but the guidelines have gradually changed. In theory at least, veterans who are using either the outpatient or the inpatient hospital facilities do not receive free care unless they are indigent, and there is a well-developed income verification system. In 1994 the Veterans Administration reported that 78 percent of those applying for care had incomes "consistent with" the data of the VA itself. This vague statement suggests that criteria may vary according to circumstances and political pressures.

The Veterans Administration hospitals are, relatively speaking, well funded. Admission to them is available to all with service-connected disabilities, but for other veterans, admission, particularly for long stays, is negotiable, based on a combination of factors, which include the applicant's financial status, the availability of beds, and the current state of funding. The quality of care in general is very good.

In 1994 there were 172 medical centers, each with a hospital and an outpatient facility. In addition there were 128 nursing-care units and 193 other outpatient units. They totalled over 75,000 beds, 79 percent of which were occupied in 1994 by veterans whose ailments

79

are not connected with their military service in most cases. There were over a million patients treated in the hospitals in 1994, and 25 million in the outpatient clinics. The total outlay for this was $15.4 billion.

Veterans Administration medical facilities offer a complete range of medical services and ancillary support services, as well as carry out a vigorous research program that has produced some widely acclaimed studies. Many of the Veterans Administration hospitals are affiliated with medical schools, helping to train thousands of American doctors. Some of these hospitals also train interns and residents.

Over the years, suggestions have been made that veterans' care be integrated into the general medical system for which the civilian hospitals and clinics would be reimbursed. One of President Nixon's long-range goals was to separate the federal government from all direct medical care. On a small scale this has been going on for several years under the CHAMPUS Program for service personnel for whom the nearest federal facility is not available or otherwise suitable.

People who are veterans and who wish to use one of these medical services can find the details for applying from their local veterans' agent or by calling the nearest VA facility.

OTHER HEALTH-CARE DELIVERY SYSTEMS

Other health-care delivery systems exist as well. Some unions operate clinics for their members. An extensive program of inpatient and ambulatory care established by the United Mineworkers after World War II proved too costly for the union. Many large industrial and business companies offer daytime weekday services, even checkups, as well as attention to immediate medical problems on-site. Insurance companies in many cities have established clinics for the treatment of work-related ailments. Industrial medicine is a subspecialty in and of itself with its own journals, professional society, and professional meetings. Close and confidential doctor-patient relationships seldom develop under circumstances where the third party paying for the services of nurses and physicians is not primarily representing the interests of the patient.

COLLEGE HEALTH CARE

Colleges and universities generally offer insurance for prepaid care, which is often quite comprehensive. The care ranges from nurse-run daytime sick call with limited hours, to a full service complete with sophisticated infirmary care and a staff of specialists, both usually available only to students. Several large universities also offer care to faculty, employees, and even to dependents. The American College Health Association through its journal and annual medical conventions, has contributed to the increased professionalism and competence among college health personnel. To the extent that the college nurses and doctors are seen as respecting confidentiality, and having the patients' interests at heart, they can successfully overcome some of the students' problems relating to authority figures.

ARMED FORCES HEALTH CARE

The armed forces also offer comprehensive prepaid inpatient and outpatient (ambulatory) care to eligible service personnel and their dependents. There are military medical journals, a first-rate medical school, and professional societies of military physicians. The care is usually of high quality, if somewhat lacking in continuity of personalized care. As in the case of students and their college health services, doctors and nurses in the military must overcome the skeptical stereotypes of some service personnel.

CLINICS FOR WOMEN

Special clinics exist also for women's health, providing routine gynecological exams, reproductive counseling, and contraceptive and abortion services. Most managed-care plans provide these services, but some women prefer the anonymity and confidentiality of an entirely separate medical record and encounter. Private and sometimes public funds provide support when the fees women can afford are insufficient to cover the costs of the service. Managed-care plans do not pay for such visits, as they control costs by using their own doctors and nurses. At present, some politicians have brought to the issue of public funding for reproductive health care the strong emotions surrounding the abortion issue, and in the buildup to the 1996 elections more attacks, both verbal and physical, threaten the existence of these clinics. Their staffs may expect further harassment, but despite difficult and sometimes dangerous working conditions most have stayed the course. Planned Parenthood, long a resource for women, is trying to buck the trend of political correctness by continuing its programs of reproductive education and by continuing to support the clinics that are under siege. The future is not clear, and the financing of women's health-care clinics will continue to be a struggle.

SUBSTANCE ABUSE TREATMENT CENTERS

Addiction is a social as well as medical problem. Addiction treatment centers may exist as independent clinics or as parts of hospitals.

Alcohol abuse is a more pervasive and destructive force in this country than is drug abuse. Hospitalization for alcoholics is often a necessary first step in efforts to achieve lasting sobriety. The necessary length of time for treatment is a matter of debate. Financial consultants, of course, favor a short-term, five- to ten-day regime. Programs such as the much-admired one in Hazelden, Minnesota, favor a minimum of thirty or even sixty days, and in some instances several months. If we consider alcoholism a straightforward disease process, then we might expect a health-care plan to pay for hospital care, as some do, for a limited period of time. Other plans do not pay at all, on the grounds that alcoholism is not simply a medical disease but a complex, all-enveloping, and socially destructive obsession. Under these circumstances it is reasonable to look for public (that is, tax) support for treatment, much as in the treatment of narcotic addiction and criminal behavior.

Methadone maintenance clinics in urban centers serve thousands of addicts every year, keeping them from the illegal heroin market and in many cases enabling them to continue to function as family members and taxpayers, although the operation as well as the basic concept of these clinics has its detractors. Admission to a methadone maintenance program follows careful screening for appropriateness of this approach, after consideration of past behaviors. Admission to such a program is voluntary. Patients can be self-referred or recommended by a parole officer or social worker. Federal money provides most of the support of methadone maintenance clinics. Those admitted to such programs require close monitoring. Communities usually resist the establishment of new methadone clinics, and many authorities still object to the concept of providing narcotics to addicts, many of whom have criminal records. The authorities who run the methadone programs, on the other hand, claim that the public is protected and the costs to society are less than those that would be incurred were these people allowed to go on with use of illegal drugs.

THE TELEPHONE CALL AND THE HOUSE CALL

Last, but by no means least, in any thinking about the delivery of health care must be two of the traditional mainstays of good practice—the telephone call and, an almost forgotten medical transaction, the house call. Most managed-care plans try to have their nurses and doctors use the telephone frequently to give diagnoses and advice, which forestall the need for an office visit. But a very good case can also be made for the cost savings of the house call under certain circumstances.

Most family doctors and almost all pediatricians and their well-trained assistants can, and do, make diagnoses and prescribe treatments over the telephone. The success of this transaction depends on mutual trust, the competence of the professional, and the severity of the condition. Mistakes can, of course, occur. Some patients or parents cannot be reassured except by a face-to-face visit with the doctor. In most instances, however, the diagnoses and treatment are satisfactory, the family is reassured, and everyone has saved time and money. The downside of this method is the open invitation it presents to those inclined to initiate malpractice litigation. The primary-care practitioner is at considerable risk. As medical records are an essential part of quality control, the doctor or nurse who gives the telephone advice or prescription should make a note for the patient's record. A careful managed-care plan might be well advised to have its caregivers record each such call and transcribe it into the record, even though by doing so they would be going against policy by incurring extra costs.

Lawyers routinely record and time every telephone call, adding up their "billable hours," and this is a well-accepted procedure. Few physicians charge for calls; if they did they might find the burden of answering from twenty to fifty or more calls a day easier to bear. They would also be more willing to dispense advice in a timely and humane manner. From time to time an understanding patient who has received a lot of telephone advice and prescribing will ask the doctor to bill him for the calls. The astonished doctor, I know from personal experience, is grateful for this recognition.

There is another side to the use of the phone by doctors. The telephone can also be an unwelcome intruder on a busy schedule.

Which is worse for the patient, to be interrupted and to wait in the doctor's office while he or she answers calls, or to be on the outside repeatedly calling the doctor's office and awaiting a return call? There is no good answer to this question. The physician's receptionist is also in a difficult situation. He or she is supposed to be a gatekeeper while at the same time a sympathetic and reassuring listener, interrupting the doctor only for a matter of extreme urgency.

Alexander Graham Bell may have revolutionized the practice of medicine, but he made it much more complicated for doctors. The fact that an electrocardiogram or cardiac monitor recording can be transmitted to a specialist center over the telephone wire is one compensatory benefit, and the fax is on its way to replacing mailed written reports. Yet many people may have the opportunity to see a fax on its way between the sender and the recipient, just as other people may find a way to overhear a highly confidential telephone call.

The house call has almost disappeared, for reasons that are not altogether persuasive. It takes more time than an office call, sophisticated equipment is not available, and usually no colleague or assistant is on hand for consultation. These are valid objections, but there are some circumstances in which the house call is better medical practice as well as cheaper for the patient. For example, an elderly couple with no automobile need to have their chronic congestive heart failure and blood pressure checked at regular intervals as well as to be checked for the possible early symptoms of Parkinson's disease or Alzheimer's disease. These determinations can be made simply, by the use of eyes, ears, stethoscope, blood pressure cuff, and, above all, a primary-care practitioner's brain.

I have found that some older people, nervous in the doctor's office, have the appearance of a borderline elevation of blood pressure. A house call by the doctor or nurse practitioner under relaxed circumstances often produces a "cure" of this hypertension. The physician can make the call at a convenient time (such as on the way to or from work). The telephone does not interrupt. The doctor can see at a glance around the house telltale signs of deterioration, of incapacity, of depression. He or she can quickly see the medicine or liquor bottles, the food supply, the obstacles to living such as steep stairs, lack of heat, or electrical hazards. All this can be done in ten minutes or less. The patients are satisfied, and the doctor knows a lot more about the patients and how they live. At the same time, there is no worry about transportation or a long wait for the patients in the doctor's office. The doctor has to drive and park to be sure (remembering that he or she is on the way home anyway), and perhaps he or she does not really need the tea and cakes the grateful patients offer. On the way home, the doctor can then dictate the clinical notes and instructions for the office file.

How would the managed-care "bean counters" assess the monetary value of this doctor's service? Is it worth as much as two office calls? If the patients came to the office, might not he have ordered some expensive laboratory work or X rays, which he would not have ordered if the patient stayed at home?

Once on a house call to a woman subject to severe migraine headaches, I saw that there were three normal, lively children, yet the house was painfully neat and the children strictly controlled. This brief encounter revealed a lot about what was behind the woman's migraines.

To take another example: a single mother is at home with three young children; one has a sore throat and an earache. The nurse practitioner could come by taxi or by car, examine and prescribe. The savings in time and anxiety and family disruption have no easily assessed monetary value. The managed-care plan does not have to pay the babysitter and taxi fare for the mother and child because the mother must do so. Of course, an office visit costs the plan less than sending the nurse, so the plan can boast how it has cut costs. The costs, however, exist—only the payment is made by the consumer. In the language of business, this is known as cost-shifting, and it is thought to be an acceptable strategy.

Nurse practitioners, often associated with a Visiting Nurse Association, do make house calls on request by a doctor. The fee is covered by Medicare or other insurance plans. A group practice or health-care plan may send out nurse practitioners to make an assessment and report back as to the need for laboratory studies, X rays, or hospitalization. In other cases, in some states, nurse practitioners can make these calls independently, as primary-care providers. In effect, they are private practitioners. In some cities there are now available independent organizations, listed in the Yellow Pages, that will, on request, supply doctors for calls to hotels or homes, usually on a strictly cash basis.

The list of other agencies coping with health-care needs is impressive. For example, the 1995 *Human Services Yellow Pages* for the Boston area lists over 18,000 human services available in Massachusetts and Rhode Island alone. Included are almost all public and private facilities. For someone seeking help, a managed-care plan can also be a wonderful resource; for others who are not in a plan, the Internet may prove to be a boon.

Some Trends in Health-Care Delivery

Computerization of patient data will soon be the dominant method of record keeping. It is already preferred because of the ease of communication of essential data, legibility, quick retrieval, and the ability to check the patient's records against protocols or practice guidelines for quality-assurance purposes, thereby protecting the patient. An article in the American College of Physicians', *Observer* said, "A quiet revolution is taking place which promises to change the way physicians get information from hospitals, payers, and related organizations." At present about 40 percent of physicians in all specialties have access to a database, according to BMI Medical Information, Inc.; soon almost all doctors will use computers.

There are also networks giving medical information of all sorts. For example, subscribers to the American College of Physicians network pay only $4 a month. Subscribing physicians receive periodic updates, and can request references and position papers. The world's largest on-line network is CompuServe, and now medical information on the Internet is available through this service. A computer carried by a doctor "covering" for others on nights and holidays can provide access to needed information concerning patients, but for the private practitioner the costs of such access can be high. A full practice-management package (computer, modem, software, and access to on-line information) can cost up to $10,000, according to the American College of Physicians.

Another type of information source is typified by CHINS, the Community Health Information Network, which makes instantly available laboratory and X-ray reports. A similar application is at work at St. Vincent's Health Center in Jacksonville, Florida, serving 200 physicians practicing in that area who are on the hospital staff. Each physician is equipped with a modem and the system software.

Errors in prescribing and administration of medication have been heavily publicized. One world-famous and respected cancer hospital in Boston faced a lawsuit and governmental censure for such an occurrence in 1995. Studies of such hospital mishaps show that one reason why the system fails is that many different medicines are being prescribed by several different doctors. Modern specialty care can result in one doctor not knowing which other doctors have seen the patient and what they have done. Such errors are more easily detected by matching the computer record of the prescription to a standard protocol that lists the patient's known allergies and physical findings. More and more pharmacies computerize prescriptions, and the patient's medications are then automatically screened for errors in dosage or compatibility. I have had reason on several occasions to be grateful to a pharmacist who has called me about such matters, including the fact that the patient had gotten prescriptions from other doctors without telling me.

An unfortunate aspect of computerization of medical information is the loss of confidentiality, much as its proponents deny it. There are too many possibilities for unauthorized, often-unwitting dissemination of a patient's private data. In fact, the idea is now widespread among physicians and many of their patients who are familiar with computerization that medical confidentiality is relative, not absolute. Many HMOs, to their credit, are making heroic efforts to prevent "leaks." The Harvard Community Health Plan in 1995 tightened access to patient information and announced restrictions on the recording of some sensitive material in physicians' notes onto computer, particularly matters discussed with psychotherapists.

Quality of Health Care

Everyone wants good quality in health care. Since no one could be against high quality, why should there be a problem? The answer lies in the definition. An eminent judge faced with another difficult definition said of pornography, "I can't define it, but I know it when I see it." So it is with the quality of health care. A great teaching hospital announces a great research breakthrough; that sounds like quality. But when a patient in that same hospital cannot seem to get any attention from a nurse or a doctor, that does not sound like quality. The quality of care rendered by a highly trained specialist in a particular field is the universal ideal. Under managed care, generalists are under pressure to treat patients in some of these specialized fields without referral; this places the generalist in a vulnerable position.

As Dr. Fred Rosner of the Mt. Sinai School of Medicine in New York wrote in 1995, "Good primary care internists, pediatricians, and family practitioners are being forced to take on the role of being mediocre specialists. . . . The term managed care is an oxymoron, since 'care' requires flexibility and judgment, whereas 'managed' implies rigidity and rules." While the generalist can achieve some protection by following practice guidelines laid down by the organizations, the resulting care may not be to the satisfaction of either the doctor or the patient. This topic will be debated for years, probably without any consensus being reached. Naturally every person wants the most expert care for him- or herself and for family members and friends. Practice guidelines have been established that outline the principles of care for many conditions, with the usually accepted course of management and treatment. Following the guidelines is not usually mandatory, but the physician or nurse who operates outside of them invites criticism and possible disciplinary action.

Satisfaction with quality of care is subjective, so ongoing studies of health-care options can only give general conclusions. Some people like and trust their doctor without reservation. To them that represents quality health care (without questioning the doctor's up-to-date medical knowledge). Others judge the quality of their medical care by the academic qualifications and professional standing of their doctor, even if the doctor is cold, uncommunicative, and hard to reach. Still others judge quality of care by costs of co-payments, accessibility of care, and coverage for medical procedures that are of importance to them. Very often people find the ideal combination, but it may take much searching and trial and error. In chapters 3 (Caregivers) and 6 (Hospitals) I have suggested some criteria for judging quality, but in the end self-knowledge and knowledge of the system is the best approach.

5

Money and Costs

Although human life is priceless, we always act as if something had an even greater price than life. But what is that something?

ANTOINE DE SAINT-EXUPERY, *Night Flight*

Any sensible person wants to know the cost of anything he or she may buy, and health care should be no exception. These costs, however, may be subtle and hard to identify. Fifty years ago, the distinguished New York physician and public-health expert Dr. Haven Emerson pointed out that the "social cost of illness is incalculable." At present the actual cost in dollars of health care is also almost incalculable. Our national income in "real dollars" is falling while the expenditures on health care continue to rise. Money discussions are often confusing and at the same time boring, but not to know what you are paying and are going to pay, and what you are going to receive for your money, is a serious mistake. Unless we understand something of the factors that produce these costs, we can hardly hope to reform the system. Here is a short summary of some of the issues:

· Everyone would like the best care in both technological and humane terms. Everyone is looking for a Dr. Wonderful.
· Everyone is ambivalent about whether he or she wants to pay for that same high quality of care for him- or herself, let alone for someone else.
· Health care is expensive for each of us under any system, and it will surely become more so. All of us will pay for it either directly or in taxes, or both.
· Many academics, financiers, and politicians are trying to find ways to satisfy everyone.
· No plan or system can possibly satisfy everyone.
· Health care is a test of our national ability to cease demanding everything for ourselves and to be fair to others, even a bit generous.

Dr. Stephen A. Schroeder, president of the Robert Wood Johnson Foundation, said in his annual report for 1994: "Because the demand for medical care surely will exceed the national willingness to pay for it, the challenge of health care cost containment is likely to endure for as long as there are patients needing care, institutions in place to offer services, and the trained professionals to provide them."

In the United States we have the highest per capita spending on health care in the world. This should produce the best results, but of the eight most developed nations, we have the highest infant-mortality rate, the shortest life expectancy for men and women, and the lowest percentage of fully immunized children. In this regard we do not seem to be getting good value for our money. In 1960 we spent 5.3 percent of the gross domestic product on health care, but by 1993 this figure had risen to 13.9 percent. Our national health expenditures in 1970 were $74.4 billion, and in 1993 the amount had risen to $884 billion. The amount spent per capita on health services and supplies in 1970 was $322, and in 1993 it had reached $3,299. During this same period the expenditures for Medicare were $154 billion and for Medicaid $123 billion.

One might expect, on seeing these increases in spending for health care, that the number of people admitted to hospitals would have risen sharply during this period, but they actually fell. This is not by any means a worldwide trend: none of the other developed countries show the same drop in hospital admissions, which in this country is almost certainly primarily due to the sharp increase in ambulatory surgery as opposed to hospital admission for the same surgery. In 1980 3.2 million surgical procedures were done outside of the hospital, and in 1992 the number had risen to 12.9 million. Perhaps, one could imagine, Americans are visiting their doctors more frequently than do people in other developed countries. According to the 1994 *Statistical Abstract of the United States*, in 1992 there were 1.5 billion visits to medical facilities with a rate per person of 5.5 visits per year, but this rate represents fewer visits than in any other developed country. Of these visits for care, 834 million were in offices and clinics, and 222 million were in hospitals. Additionally, during this period it was calculated that 181 million medical contacts were completed by telephone.

A tremendous number of these health-care transactions were supported by federal taxes. In 1992 35.6 million elderly and disabled people were enrolled in Medicare, and 31.1 million "medically indigent" people were enrolled in Medicaid.

In the last twelve years, more and more people's health care was paid for by lump sum payments to HMOs. From 1980 to 1992, the number of plans rose from 236 to 5,466, and each of these plans enrolled many more people; their numbers rising from 9.1 million to 41.38 million in twelve years, and the trend is progressing faster than ever. And where are the premiums of businesses and employees going? In December of 1994 the *Wall Street Journal* reported figures on the ten largest HMOs in this country, showing that each of them has accumulated a substantial amount of cash. The largest,

United Health Care, had cash and investments of $2.6 billion. The Associated Press reported in November 1995 that United Health Care posted a profit for the year of $400 million and paid its chief executive $4 million in direct payment, exclusive of his stock holdings. When US Healthcare merged with Aetna in June 1996, the C.E.O. reportedly received personally almost a billion dollars.

Yet there are many reasons for the increase in the costs of medical care, beyond the inflation in wages and salaries and the profits paid to the health-care plans. More people demand and receive very expensive, highly technical tests of which the most conspicuous are magnetic resonance imaging (MRI), computerized axial tomography (CAT scan), ultrasound, including echocardiograms, and the use of many radioactive isotopes as tracers in diagnostic testing. More people are given treadmill stress tests, and more people are receiving coronary artery bypass grafts as well as other forms of open-heart surgery at tremendous expense. Another increase in cost comes as a result of the effective and highly specialized use of various methods of intensive care. By 1992 there were 96,707 intensive-care beds in this country, operating at a cost of $55 billion and accounting for 11.3 percent of all hospital inpatient admissions.

Third-party payment by the health insurer for obtaining a second opinion has been introduced with an eye to cutting down on some procedures, especially surgical, but as the person rendering the second opinion also has to be paid, the savings may not be as great as would first appear. Within a hospital or in a small community the doctor rendering the second opinion is often a friend and colleague of the doctor who proposes a specific procedure.

Another factor greatly contributing to the cost of health care is the rising number of patients admitted to emergency rooms in hospitals because of illness or injury related to substance abuse, alcohol, cocaine, heroin, and other drugs. The need to meet the ever-expanding requirements for procedures and standards expected of hospitals by the Joint Commission on Accreditation of Health Care

Organizations (JCAHCO), and by the hospitals' own malpractice advisors, has also made the operation of hospitals more expensive.

The costs of visits to the doctor have also risen. Physicians, as we have noted, usually have heavy indebtedness by the time they finish their training, and in addition they must pay annual premiums for malpractice insurance ranging from $5,000 to over $100,000 per year. The lowest malpractice rates go to generalists who do no surgery, no invasive procedures, and no radiation or chemotherapy. The highest rates are charged to specialists in orthopedics, plastic surgery, obstetrics, and neurosurgery. These rates also reflect wide regional variations, the highest being in some sections of Los Angeles and New York City. The insurance is charged to the individual doctor. Most managed-care plans at present try to entice doctors to join by paying these insurance premiums. Their fees need to cover these expenses as well as overhead. They must also pay for continuing education in order to maintain their hospital standing. The exponential increase in required record keeping and reporting has forced physicians and clinics to employ larger and larger staffs to handle this paperwork and accounting. Every practice requires legal advice, often at great expense, as well as accountants and billing services. Salaried doctors working in managed-care plans do not have these expenses, which are covered by the plan. In return, these doctors receive a smaller income and must maintain a high level of productivity. The costs assumed by the plan are paid for by subscribers' premiums.

Government Funding of Health-Care Services

MEDICARE

Medicare, established in 1965, was originally budgeted to be self-sustaining, with a perpetual trust fund to receive the contributions from subscribers' and employers' taxes and monthly contributions.

The monthly premium has risen over the past thirty years from about $10 to more than $40 a month. Despite this, the fund is being rapidly depleted. The General Accounting Office estimates that the fund will be bankrupt by the year 2001 unless drastic changes are made.

Medicare is divided into two parts. Part A is for hospital insurance and is designed to pay a portion of the cost for inpatient care, limited skilled-nursing-facility care, intermittent home health care, and hospice care. Part A does not cover payment for the first day of the stay, which at present costs $696. After a covered hospital stay of more than sixty days, there is a significant co-payment requirement.

Part B of Medicare is voluntary and requires payment of a premium, which in 1996 was $42.60 a month. This is usually deducted from the Social Security or Railroad Retirement check each month, as mandated by law. Part B is designed primarily to pay part of the cost for physician services, outpatient care, and durable medical equipment. There is a financial penalty if you do not sign up for Part B when you turn sixty-five. Part B has a yearly $100 deductible, and most services covered under Part B require that the patient give a 20 percent co-payment. The gaps in Medicare coverage, therefore, come from such matters as routine physical examinations, dental care, eye exams and eyeglasses, hearing aids, prescription drugs outside of the hospital, and nonskilled nursing or rest-home care. To fill in these gaps in coverage, there are many policies known colloquially as Medigap plans. These are only effective if the person already has Medicare Parts A and B. The Health Care Financing Administration (HCFA) publishes an annual guidebook entitled *The Medicare Handbook*, which answers almost every imaginable question on these topics.

MEDICAID

Medicaid is a program jointly funded by federal and state coffers for certain people with limited incomes or assets. It is available to poor women, children, and families. Medicaid is also available to supplemental security income (SSI) recipients and the elderly, blind, or disabled individuals who meet the financial requirements. People who are eligible for Medicaid do not have to purchase Medigap insurance. When they are also eligible for Medicare coverage, their premiums are covered through government funding. To qualify for Medicaid one must have a monthly income that is at present below $581 for a single person and $786 for a couple. The applicant's "accountable assets" cannot be over $2,000 for a single person and $3,000 for a couple. One way in which people with marginal income become eligible for Medicaid is to "spend down" their income. Another way is to give away the house, automobile, or other tangible assets to the children. This deliberate impoverishment seems unfair, and it is sometimes abused.

Doctors and Their Incomes

No matter how highly educated a physician may be, how hard he or she works, how long the training period has been, and how short an active doctor's earning working life may be, the income of doctors seems always to be a source of controversy and often envy. In our culture, where success and status are, for the most part, measured by money, it is difficult to say where on the scale we should place our doctors. Some doctors charge high fees because they believe that some patients think that a higher fee means a better doctor. Some other doctors think that if they make more money, they must be more important, which is demonstrably untrue. Doctors working under managed care don't establish their own fees for services. All managed-care plans try to keep the income of their physicians within bounds and tied directly to productivity.

Should a physician be paid for each service, with greater skill and training and higher academic standing commanding a higher price, and should he or she be paid more for assuming higher risks? It is almost impossible to assign a relative risk or skill for every procedure; defining and policing these risks would be an expensive procedure whose results would probably be inaccurate. The patient really has no way of judging the value of a given service, or the training, skill, or risk taking involved. The dollar cost of curing, or of suffering and dying, is not measurable.

All in all it seems probable that people with equivalent intellectual skills and hard work in other occupations such as the law, real estate, or banking, who with a shorter training time have an extra ten or twenty years of useful earning life, will at the present time make more money than their medical contemporaries. The American Medical Association in 1994, after an extensive study, calculated that physicians provide annually more than $21 billion in uncompensated care because of bad debts as well as charity care. In addition, $9.8 billion of fees billed were never paid according to an article in *Managed Care* magazine.

The practice of many managed-care plans nowadays is to pay physicians more for taking on a larger number of patients under a capitation plan, encouraging them to see more patients within a given period of time. Under capitation, as in the British National Health Service for the past fifty years, the physician is paid a flat sum annually for every patient on his or her "panel." If a doctor wishes to earn more, he or she takes on more patients, which involves leaving less time available for each visit and longer waits for appointments.

There are elaborate schemes to regulate capitation practices, but the schemes themselves seem to involve considerable expense, not to mention intrusiveness and subjectivity. One such scheme invites patients to rate their physicians in terms of the doctors' promptness, courtesy, and proficiency. Another method is to study adverse outcomes, "mistakes," and expensive complications.

To take an example of how managed-care reimbursement of doctors affects care, a board-certified internist is trained in school and in residency training to take up to an hour in a routine health appraisal (checkup). Third-party reimbursement generally restricts the payment for this service to an amount that would be paid for a checkup done by another physician in ten or fifteen minutes. The well-person checkup may be paid for only once every year or even two years. The conscientious internist is free under a managed-care plan to take up to an hour for a checkup, and many still do, but he or she will lose money under a capitation plan, or if on salary be penalized by the plan for lower productivity. It is possible, and indeed frequently happens, that some physicians with a busy practice of patients on Medicare or Medicaid can run an assembly-line type of practice and earn far more in an hour than the most highly trained internist who takes more time with each patient. Although computerized records make it somewhat easier to detect such practices, there seems to be no way of forcing uniform standards of good practice at a fair rate of compensation. Nonetheless, all internists may not suffer financially under managed care.

In a recent readjustment based on the "relative value scale" by Medicare and Medicaid, surgical specialists received an 11 percent raise, but generalists and family practitioners were kept at the same level. So much for the widely publicized encouragement of family doctors. Subsequent to this, payments to *all* physicians by government and for-profit plans have become more standardized and, in many cases, reduced. The gap between the income of generalists and specialists has biased the distribution of physicians and is the target of most efforts at health-care reform, both in the public and the private sector. As we have seen in the more-integrated system in Norway, generalists are more highly paid than specialists, the latter presumably choosing their careers primarily because of their own interests and abilities.

There are no easy answers to the problem of assigning payment to physicians. The question of how to pay physicians is an ancient one. In the works of Plato, there are frequent references to the selection, training, and pay of leaders of the state, and he often made the analogy to the training and pay of physicians. Plato's goal was to develop and support high moral and intellectual caliber. The feeling was that these leaders should be paid very well, but that there should be no relation between the physicians' income and the services rendered. In real life it has been my experience that the best doctors seem to work equally as skillfully and hard and in an equally caring way regardless of the method of payment. The rotten apple spoils the barrel, as the saying goes, and the abuse of payment by some physicians has brought a bad name and oppressive regulations to the practice of medicine.

The pay of nurses has increased in the last two decades, commensurate with the extra expense and time involved in their increased training. For physicians and nurses, specialized training brings greater income, but as noted earlier, under managed care this level of compensation may not continue to increase. It seems likely that most people considering all of these factors would like to see professionals with equivalent training, intellectual skills, and good work habits being paid more or less equally.

Ways of Controlling Costs

In health care as in industry the study of cost-effectiveness has brought about many changes and has brought about a more rational approach to many procedures. It is easier to determine that a certain new technique in manufacturing will produce the same result at less cost than it is to measure, for example, the cost savings of a routine annual physical examination, or the relation of cost to lives saved in doing uterine Pap smears or mammograms at various age levels. Nevertheless, the effort and thought that are being applied to cost issues and other topics have brought an important focus to our thinking about what constitutes good and affordable care.

It is difficult to tell which routine tests are worth paying for, but it is virtually impossible to determine the cost-effectiveness of other therapies such as mental-health treatment, acupuncture, or chiropractic. One immediate problem in the mental-health field has been the inability to demonstrate the cost-effectiveness of psychotherapy. The fact that a dollar value is difficult to assign to treatment of people who are not psychotic, is a wonderful excuse for the money managers to deny payment for mental-health services to the non-psychotic. For that matter there is no consensus that psychotherapy, if it should be reimbursed, should be the exclusive domain of M.D. psychiatrists, or Ph.D.'s, social workers, or religious workers. It is one thing to measure the days of salaried work lost by surgical repair of a hernia, but another matter altogether to determine whether behavioral treatment with transcendental meditation, yoga, and similar methods produces greater productivity as measured in dollars and cents, or whether treatments such as acupuncture, herbal medicine, and massage are cost-effective ways of treating intractable chronic conditions.

One way in which costs can be and have already been cut in many managed-care health plans and in some states is by the use of generic equivalents instead of brand-name drugs. This practice is preferred and sometimes mandated by managed-care plans. The British National Health Service, very early in its existence, found that people were using what appeared to be an excessive number of prescription medicines, eyeglasses, canes, and crutches that were free to the public, so the health service instituted a co-payment. Later, under various plans in this country that reimburse for drugs, there have been attempts to curb excessive use by various means. In 1981 the state of New Hampshire reported that for eleven months it limited the number of prescriptions reimbursable by Medicaid. A subsequent study revealed that schizophrenics who were denied more than three prescriptions per month ended up using more of the mental-health services, including frequent hospitalizations. This attempt at saving money cost the state $1,530 per patient, seventeen times the savings in drug costs. No one should be denied medications essential to their health. Modern medicines are expensive, but worth it. We need to work to control costs to the extent possible.

Several mail-order prescription services, of which perhaps the best known is operated by the American Association of Retired Persons (AARP), and many managed-care plans have an arrangement with certain pharmacies to sell prescription drugs from an approved list at below cost, or for a nominal charge, the difference being paid by the managed-care plan. Group purchasing can also bring about considerable savings. Some university health services, some union health plans, and many rural cooperatives effect substantial savings on medications through group purchase.

Most large managed-care organizations have pharmacy committees that determine the costs of medications that have equivalent action and issue formularies for their physicians to use. The pharmaceutical firms' response is to point out that the quality of generics is not always closely supervised or regulated, which is true. Many generic drugs are manufactured in Third World countries (although many of the factories are U.S. owned) with very little supervision. There is an association of generic-drug companies, but it has no regulatory powers. The proprietary drugs, on the other hand, must undergo rigorous testing by the Food and Drug Administration (FDA). As time goes on, more and more managed-care plans will contract with pharmaceutical manufacturers to supply medications for their patients at the lowest negotiable cost. As there is no FDA program to test the purity and effectiveness of generics (as opposed to brand names), the responsibility for this testing will rest with the plan.

Pharmaceutical manufacturers continue to introduce new and highly effective, but expensive, medications sometimes for conditions for which there were formerly few effective drugs, but many of the older, less-expensive medications will work just as well. Managed-care plans, the AARP, Consumer Union, and other organizations try to inform the public about their choices of medication. On the other hand, advertising stimulates customer demand for the latest remedy.

COST SHARING

In an effort to prevent overuse of medical care, insurers try to indoctrinate their subscribers with the concept of saving money. The most familiar method is co-payment, which means that at the time of the visit, the patient pays out of his or her pocket a part of the fee. Another form of cost sharing occurs in the Medicare system. Under Medicare, elderly patients are supposed to pay 20 percent of each ambulatory-care visit, or a large fee ($716 in 1995) for each hospital admission. Most people on Medicare or their employers buy supplemental insurance, such as Medex, to cover this difference. Whether this supplemental insurance is through a governmental or for-profit agency, the policy is known as Medigap insurance. This system seems difficult for most people to understand, cumbersome in operation, and expensive to administer. Confusion assails the patient who typically receives several bills, not to mention statements that are headed, "This is not a bill." Doctors' offices spend countless hours helping patients understand the system; this adds greatly to the cost of running a practice.

The need for such patients to make co-payment means that they have to be prepared to carry cash, and the doctor's office is also busy making change and handing out receipts. This form of cost sharing as a means of cutting down on supposedly inappropriate care probably does not even achieve its objective. Several studies have concluded that appropriate care (as well as inappropriate care) was equally reduced by such cost-sharing measures. In other words, people go to the doctor because they want to and feel they need to; they feel the need to go without reference to someone else's idea of what is appropriate. These studies also showed that poor people who could not afford to pay for coinsurance received less medical care and had fewer mammograms and Pap smears.

RATIONING

More than half of our health-care expenditures pay for services delivered in the last six months of a patient's life and in the treatment of incurable illnesses. As a consequence, in many countries over the last fifty years, the idea that this is a place to cut expenses has received wide support. It is, and probably will be for the foreseeable future, one of the most hotly debated topics in medical care. The healthy young person paying a lot for health care in cash and in taxes may feel one way; the families of an elderly person who is slowly but surely declining may feel otherwise.

"The specter of medical rationing—the deliberate withholding of potentially beneficial care—is usually involved in health care policy discussion as a dreaded consequence of either the containment of soaring medical expenditures or the expansion of health insurance coverage," says Dr. Stephen A. Schroeder, president of the Robert Wood Johnson Foundation. He goes on to point out that rationing does in fact exist in every country, but that in America it is only implicit: managed-care plans limit certain services partially or wholly, and their physicians are under surveillance by the plan or agency that pays them.

Some treatments, such as bone-marrow transplantation for leukemia, were, for a time, considered to be experimental by insurers and therefore not covered. In most cases this is now an accepted treatment, and the estimated cost is $140,000 per transplantation. Litigation often arises over coverage for less-established procedures. Expensive treatments for the elderly that might not be paid for in Germany, Britain, or Sweden, usually considered to be welfare states, are paradoxically more commonly carried out and paid for in this country through Medicare. Indigent and disabled Americans frequently receive expensive care through Medicare or Medicaid that would not be paid for in any other country. For example, in Britain there are age limits above which the National Health Service will not pay for kidney, heart, or other organ transplants. Our Medicare system does not deny payments for any procedure because of age. In practice, however, as Dr. Schroeder implies, hospitals as well as doctors are reluctant to carry out heroic, high-technology procedures on the old and infirm. Utilization reviews and quality-assurance reviews, which are widely carried out by hospitals and by managed-care plans, may question the appropriateness of such operations. It will require much persuasion by political leaders to get such organizations as the AARP and groups of the disabled to accept cuts in such benefits. There does not seem to be much popular support in European countries for adopting the American model of total health-care services for those over sixty-five years of age.

Even if you have "full coverage" within your managed-care plan, there may be buried in the small print information about limits beyond which the plan will not pay. This is known as a "cap." The figure for the cap may seem absurdly high, but there are some extremely expensive illnesses. AIDS, hemophilia, automobile accidents, and in some cases multiple sclerosis come to mind. Be sure you know about any cap on your coverage. It is possible to buy supplemental "disaster" insurance to cover costs that exceed the cap.

There will always be a few people in this world who can afford any medical care they want. A for-profit hospital, in fact, was built within this decade with American capital in Scotland, including the latest in technological equipment and employing highly paid specialists. Rumor has it that the investors misjudged the market and that sick rich people are going elsewhere. In the United States high-quality, fee-for-service care is legal and still widely available, although such care may become restricted in the next decade in deference to the traditional liberal American espousal of egalitarianism or equal access to care for everyone. Equal care and equal access to care are not at present the norm. Famous celebrities who are athletes, congressmen, and entertainers seem to be able to "check in" to hospitals at will, according to media reports. Organs for liver or heart transplants, available to many people only after a very long wait, if ever, seem to materialize suddenly for some of the rich and famous.

Hospital Costs

Everyone is appalled by the rapid increase in hospital costs. According to the U.S. Department of Commerce, in 1992 costs in community hospitals reached $820 per day or $5,794 for the average stay. During this time, interestingly enough, fewer people were hospitalized than in previous decades. There were 147 admissions per thousand patients in 1972, and only 122 per thousand in 1992. Much of the drop came about because of the rise in day surgery, and even more because of the strict governmental utilization review standards governing hospital admissions. Under the rapidly spreading system called capitation, in which doctors and hospitals receive preset sums to provide all care to groups of people, hospitals must not only slash costs but also redirect their goals. The costs of care before and after the surgery have been lifted from the shoulders of the managed-care or insurance plan and placed squarely on the family, who must bring the patient to and from home and do the home care necessitated by the surgery. No one has figures for the financial and emotional costs to the patient and his or her family of this cost saving.

As a result of the decrease in hospitalization rates, all hospitals have empty beds. Community hospitals are costly, quite frequently losing money, but teaching hospitals cost even more, and they are losing money even faster. One reason is that teaching hospitals do 44 percent of all the free care in the United States, caring for the sickest people while possessing only 18 percent of all American acute-care beds. Managed-care plans are negotiating with teaching hospitals, striving to achieve a financial deal that is the best for the insurer. Teaching hospitals are required by government regulation to give a certain amount of free care. This amount is fixed by a complicated formula and by negotiation. If, in addition to this, such hospitals accept from managed-care plans payments arrived at by underbidding other hospitals, their financial woes are made even worse. Teaching hospitals are now competing with each other for their share of the pool of the managed-care patients and with the community hospitals for these admissions. Managed-care plans, therefore, are in a strong bargaining position. Teaching hospitals are reducing the size of their staffs and the services offered.

As a result of problems with teaching hospitals, the education and training of young doctors, nurses, and all other health-care workers is already suffering and will surely suffer further. Internships (the first year of residency training) and residencies (years two to five of postgraduate training) have already been cut by 20 percent. Soon there will not be enough training slots available for our U.S. medical-school graduates. Inevitably, our medical schools will admit fewer students. The trend has already begun.

Funding Research and Education

The extraordinary growth of biomedical research in the past fifty years has already produced wonderful payoffs in the diagnosis and treatment of disease. Unfortunately, these advances are not reflected in a drop in the numbers of deaths due to serious illness in this country when compared with other developed nations, partly because we have not been willing to pay for medical care for all, or even for general preventive measures. Most research has been paid for out of tax revenues; these dollars will be vastly reduced in the next few years. Medical schools, universities, and teaching hospitals have added some of their own money, in fact all they can afford, to the total support of research. Private industry is the only growing source of support for research, because of the profits that can be made by the introduction of new technologies and drugs. Part of the cost of medical education also comes from medical schools' research funding, and much of the increased cost of teaching-hospital care is related to research activities. Research grants, led by the National Institutes of Health (NIH) have up to now been giving generous allowances for "overhead," up to 50 percent over the cost of the researchers' salary, equipment, and supplies. The teaching hospitals depend on this overhead for a large part of their operating expenses. The research workers are not only permitted, but expected, to spend some time teaching the medical students and residents, at no cost to the hospital. Teaching hospitals must make classroom and teaching aids available. Usually many administrators on the hospital payroll oversee contracts, monitor expenses, and try to coordinate the activities of teaching and research with patient care. To separate out the cost of all these functions is almost impossible; the boundaries are blurred. When fewer research workers are available in teaching hospitals, either students and residents will get less teaching and supervision, or other sources of pay will need to be developed. At this time no one seems to have a workable plan for supporting the research that must be carried out if this country is to continue its preeminence in medical advances.

Many valiant efforts by the government and private foundations to separate the costs of education and research from the actual costs of delivery of direct medical care have not brought about any substantial changes. For example, more than half of medical-student teaching is done by residents, or full-time staff members, or research fellows, whose work is paid for in part by higher hospital rates. These same fellows derive most of their income from government grants for doing research "full time." The direct support of medical schools by the federal government fell from 71 percent of the schools' total income in 1964 to 38 percent in 1990. Medical educators, through the Association of American Medical Colleges, and in the pages of the journal *Academic Medicine*, have generally reported feeling that if teaching and research were separately supported, the total appropriations to medical schools would be reduced.

A popular argument goes that patients in teaching hospitals should pay more because they are getting better care. The truth of such an assertion cannot be proved by statistics. The teaching-hospital people say that their patients are sicker as a group, and this seems to be true. Teaching hospitals, as we have said, care for a disproportionate number of the seriously ill urban poor. They also have referred to them the more obscure and costly-to-treat illnesses, and at the same time they use the most advanced technology. Before taking sides, or proposing drastic solutions, we need to be aware of and think about these factors in planning any health-care "reform." Medical education is long, hard, and expensive, and nursing training has also become longer, more difficult, and more expensive. We cannot afford to withdraw support from research or training either, if we wish to continue as the world leader in medicine.

In a perfect world we would admit the best and brightest to medical school and pay all of their tuition and living expenses until they finished their training. In return each one would be expected to spend one day a week or several weeks a year in some form of public service, patient care, or even research. With such a system in place we would have fewer problems in recruiting able, competent physicians for our underserved areas, such as inner-city clinics, rural areas, mental hospitals, nursing homes, and prisons. But this is not a perfect world, and we will probably continue to tinker with subsidizing medical education and inadequately subsidizing patients and facilities in these underserved areas.

The actual cost of educating a medical student is surprisingly hard to estimate, as most of the preclinical teaching is done in laboratories or hospital settings by full-time research workers, service chiefs, and residents. One study done recently tracked some medical students over a period of a year, estimating the cost in salary of the time actually spent by each teacher. The resulting figure for instruction alone was only around $8,000 a year. Tuitions vary greatly, being lower in state-supported schools, but the costs are in the range of from $5,000 a year to $25,000 a year, excluding living expenses. Tuition, in fact, is a relatively small part of medical school budgets now. One or two of the better-known private medical schools have even considered giving up tuition altogether. Their reasoning is that since tuition represents a small proportion of the school's total income, and loans and scholarship funds already largely supplement the students' payments, if tuition were no longer charged, low-income applicants would apply on an equal footing. The public might be thus persuaded to contribute more for medical-school scholarships.

A Single-Payer System

Physicians and health-care facilities in this country at this time are compensated from a bewildering variety of sources. There is direct cash, paying by check following receipt of a bill, payment by a nonprofit insurance company, payment by a for-profit insurance company or HMO, and payment by the federal government through Medicare or Medicaid. Under the increasingly popular capitation plans, the physician receives a flat monthly fee for each patient, whether or not he or she rendered service to that person during the given period.

As noted, there are at present 1,100 companies offering health insurance in this country, and there is no universally accepted form of billing or method of payment. The confusion of the patient and the cost to the providers is great. I believe that the money spent by various insurers in promoting their product and operating a complex system of collecting money would be better applied to reducing the cost of care. Why, therefore, should there be such resistance to the idea of all payment coming through a single mechanism? The chief answer is that the obvious single payer would be the federal government, and sentiment is running strong at this time against giving that body any more power. Perhaps a consortium of insurers could work with government to construct a simpler system of payment, with a mechanism by which the for-profit sector and the government would each have representation. In our neighbor to the north, Canada, the single-payer system has been in effect for a considerable period of time. In addition to the funds from direct-income taxation, individuals, employers, government agencies, and insurers all contribute to the pool of money, with the payment to doctors or hospitals coming from this single source in a uniform fashion. This system has its detractors, but its objective seems the most logical. The opposition in this country to the proposal to adopt this payer system is strong, motivated at least in part by those now profiting from the status quo. Canadian citizens in general like the system but deplore the taxes. Canadian doctors seem to be divided in their appraisal of their health-care system. As far as the general public is concerned, the benefits to be obtained would be seen in the simplicity of the system and the probable economy. The downside, of course, would be the possibility for manipulation of the details of operation and confusion in a politically sensitive bureaucracy. Even so, I believe we must have a single-payer system.

All of the preceding discussion refers to health-care coverage within the conventional system. When we consider that Americans spend almost as much on alternative, or unconventional health care, which is not at present reimbursed by most insurers or health plans, one can understand the reason for one of the current provisions before the Congress, which is to get the government out of the details of administering health-care payments by giving each person a lump-sum allowance. Under such a plan people could buy their own type of health care according to their needs and wishes. Unfortunately, the possibilities for abuse under such a system would seem to be at least as great as those in any other system now in existence.

6

Hospitals

Hospitals are the temples of medicine.

HENRY E. SIGERIST

Originally, hospitals in this country consisted of open wards that were intended for the homeless and the destitute. Most of the patients were seriously ill or dying. Those who could afford the cost were cared for in their own homes or in private nursing homes. Over the past hundred years, hospitals have offered increasingly sophisticated services, of high quality, to all who could afford them. There was no gatekeeping based on diagnosis. Many people went to a hospital for testing or merely for "a rest." Only serious illnesses result in hospitalization today. The major diagnoses on discharge from American hospitals are, in order: heart disease, cancer, pneumonia, fracture, and psychosis. The homeless, the destitute, and the uninsured may find that only large urban general hospitals will accept them.

Hospitals range from tiny rural facilities with no resident doctors and very few nurses to large metropolitan institutions with budgets in the hundreds of millions of dollars and a huge staff of administrators, doctors, nurses, lawyers, paraprofessional aides, technologists, maintenance people, and increasingly large numbers of security personnel. The capabilities and comprehensiveness, even the quality of hospital services, vary greatly from one hospital to another. Because of this variety, hospitals cannot be considered as a coherent whole. The American Hospital Association (which has a powerful lobbying arm that works to protect the interests of hospitals and to seek government funding) offers a variety of services to its members and monitors standards, trends, and costs.

Tax exemptions for nonprofit public hospitals were originally intended to support them for the welfare of the public, especially the poor. Most big-city nonprofit hospitals, of which perhaps the most famous is Bellevue in New York City, take care of all who come to their doors, under tremendously stressful circumstances. However, at present more and more "public" hospitals are coming under the ownership of for-profit corporations, as communities and private donors can no longer be counted on to help cover their increasing deficits. Hospitals operated for profit must pay taxes as do all other businesses. To remain profitable they must place stern limits on the number of hospital admissions, the length of stay, specialty consultations, expensive surgery, and expensive equipment, and as a result patients and physicians have less and less authority in making these decisions. Charity and generosity at times seem to be mostly of historical interest in some of our larger hospitals, although many volunteers and paid caregivers still carry on the ancient and respected traditions of caring and service.

Picking a Hospital

In a large community, if you are in a health plan with some flexibility, you may have a choice of hospitals. If you live in a small community, or if you are in a tightly restricted managed-care plan, you may have no choice. Of course, in the event of a serious emergency when you are away from home, you may be taken to the nearest hospital used by a particular police department or ambulance service. Almost all health plans will pay for emergency treatment outside their system, but they often question the true nature of the emergency, and whether going to an outside hospital was more a matter of convenience than of medical necessity. The primary-care physician's approval for an emergency room visit is required by most plans. This depends, of course, on the physician being immediately available twenty-four hours a day, which is an unlikely situation. In any case, it is important to try to find out in advance as much as you can about your plan's policies and procedures related to hospitalization.

Before selecting a hospital, do some research and ask questions about the hospital's reputation in the community and within the profession. At a minimum it should be accredited by the Joint Commission on Accreditation of Health Care Organizations (JCAHCO). Such information should be readily obtainable at the hospital or in your local public library. The details of regulatory and JCAHCO inspection reports may, under some circumstances, be open to the public, and there is increasing pressure to make them available. Some states now mandate disclosure of these reports to the public. In any case do not hesitate to ask to see them. There are now standards for training and specialty board certification in emergency care, so it would be well for you to ascertain the qualifications of the emergency staff of your hospital. Every hospital has a file with these data; usually the hospital is pleased to publicize the training and special expertise of its staff members.

Neighbors and friends who have lived in the community for a long time give useful and sometimes surprising tips. The state or county medical society, listed in your local telephone book, can give figures on the hospital size, bed capacity, services rendered, and the qualifications of the staff. Most state health departments also rate hospitals and may give out information on disciplinary actions and other statistics. Best of all, if you know a doctor in the community, ask him or her. Here are some other questions you should look into:

- Is the hospital staff open to any doctor in the community? Or is it closed? In a closed-staff system you must be a patient of a staff doctor in order to be admitted.
- How accessible is the facility by public transportation or automobile?
- If you have no doctor, or if your doctor is not on the staff, will the hospital assign one to you?

Some other things may influence your choice of a hospital such as:

- What is their policy on access to your records?
- Is there an ombudsman or other person such as a case manager to whom you can turn to appeal such arbitrary decisions as length of stay?
- Who makes the final decision on matters you may appeal?
- What assurances do you have of confidentiality?

A teaching hospital is one that has an approved residency training program. Most of them have a medical-school connection. Here you can be reasonably sure the staff members will be well trained, board-certified specialists, and the equipment and procedures will be up-to-date. Against this it must be said that the comfort of the patient is often not the first consideration in such hospitals, and responsibility for your care tends to be divided. In some of the best, however, not only is a staff member identified as your own doctor, but there is a case manager trained perhaps as a social worker or nurse, whose responsibility it is to see that all aspects of your care receive attention from admission to discharge.

The case-manager plan is also gaining favor in many nonteaching and for-profit hospitals, because less time is lost waiting for tests, and important details are less apt to be overlooked. The case manager can look at the hospital order book, and try to arrange all procedures in a rapid, orderly sequence, including specialist referrals, discharge planning, and arrangements for home follow-up. A case manager is a person employed by the hospital or HMO, frequently an R.N. who has had some training in the organization of medical care, the flow of testing procedures, the arrangements for transportation for surgery or specialized testing, and the maintenance of charts and records. She or he gives no direct care. The case manager can be your ally and friend, communicating with doctors and nurses, although he or she is not allowed to order tests or medications. Not only does the patient thereby get better care, but the hospital saves money by shortening the length of stay and by avoiding the need to cancel and reschedule conflicting test and procedure times. Nonetheless, a doctor who has always been the sole arbiter of the patient's hospital management sometimes has trouble adjusting to this new system.

In smaller hospitals, some services may be contracted separately and run for profit, for example, the emergency room, laboratory, anesthesia services, physical therapy, and the pharmacy. It may be hard for you to find out about which services are subcontracted, but you need to know, because the quality as well as the course of your care is at stake. The administrative office of the hospital has this information and ought not to refuse to disclose such arrangements. This is not to automatically condemn privatization, but a warning to be vigilant.

What to Expect When You Go to the Hospital

Admission to the hospital is not automatic. The days of going to the hospital on your own initiative and expecting to be admitted are long gone. Assuming that your physician, or your health-plan administrator, or an emergency facility has arranged for the hospital admitting office to accept you, a number of things will happen— some unavoidable.

First, you will wait your turn to be interviewed by an admitting officer, who usually is not a nurse or a doctor. Every one of the many questions to be answered were created by someone at some time to satisfy the law, the JCAHCO, the insurance companies, the police, the legislature, or the hospital staff. You have to answer all of them. Some of the more enlightened HMOs or managed-care programs can now transfer this data, which they already have, electronically to the hospital, saving you and the hospital time. Your visit to the admitting office may therefore involve much time, or it may be mercifully brief.

You may ask at this point if you can have a single room, and if you are lucky you will get it. (One secret is to have a highly contagious disease or to be obstreperous, but I cannot recommend this as a standard procedure.) Intensive-care units and recovery rooms need to have patients in one large, only partly partitioned area where the nurses can keep a close watch. Otherwise, the two-, three-, or four-bed room exists only for economy of construction and maintenance.

Usually before going to your room you are taken to have more tests of your blood, your urine, often a chest X ray, and a cardiogram. Only in a few well-integrated systems can you avoid these tests, even if you protest that these have already been done recently. The hospital in reply will protest that it has to protect itself from possible litigation or charges of negligence, even though this duplication of services costs everyone time and money. Often these tests are mandated by the JCAHCO or government agencies.

A problem often arises when people are admitted on the day of planned elective surgery and proceed to the laboratory for testing. If any of these tests are not normal, out goes the patient, the surgery is canceled, and an orgy of rescheduling takes place. Pretesting a few days before admission is usually the remedy to this situation, but the informed patient must set this up in advance. It is hard sometimes to understand the regulations, and harder still to have them waived.

After the questions are all answered, the admitting officer calls an orderly or aide to conduct you to your room, after giving you papers outlining the hospital's rules and procedures. You may be compelled to ride in a wheelchair even though you are capable of walking.

You get settled in your bed. If you are in a teaching hospital you will first be interviewed and briefly examined by a nurse. Next, a social worker will come to ask about home arrangements after discharge; the rules mandate that discharge planning start on day one. Then someone comes to see if you want the television connected (have some cash on hand). Someone else asks if you want a newspaper (more cash needed). Then the most junior physician comes to do a history and physical examination; this is either a senior medical student or a first-year intern, sometimes both. Next, a senior resident visits, then the doctor in charge of your case. Finally, there is the teaching "ward attending" for that month. Within twenty-four hours you can also expect a visit from the hospital chaplain, who may or may not suit your taste but is frequently a very great comfort and a person who will take time to answer some of your many questions.

Your own primary-care generalist may or may not have hospital admitting privileges with the power to write orders. Increasingly, generalists are strongly restricted by staff regulations as to what procedures they can order or what diagnoses they can make, within their competence. This is a trade-off: you lose the continuity and empathy, but you can be more sure of modern, competent, tertiary care. This widely used term implies acute, constant supervision, specialty consultation, and all needed equipment. The most advanced technical procedures are best carried out by younger, recently trained, full-time specialists. Under the best circumstances, your own doctor will work with them, although he or she is not paid to do so. If your primary-care doctor comes to see you in the hospital, he or she usually receives no money for the visit, but the bond between you is strengthened.

In smaller, nonteaching hospitals, patients generally have their own doctors who are responsible for doing the admission workup, making daily visits, and keeping progress notes. You may not see much of the doctor in charge of your case every day, but invariably he or she is spending more time with charts, orders, telephone consultations, and visits to the X-ray department than at your bedside. Somehow it is hard for the doctor to convey to the patient the time and effort involved; to the patient, the hurried daily bedside visit may not seem enough to warrant the charges.

You have filled out the menu for the next day and look forward to this attractive-sounding break in the day's routine. In most cases the food purchased is of high quality, and the menu is scientifically planned. Somehow, between the kitchen and your bedside, it loses its appeal. Sick people, particularly those with pain, fever, or under sedative medications, have little appetite and little energy to consume a meal. Hospital food is a leading cause of complaints and a favorite butt of jokes. Even so, it is generally superior to economy-class airline food, to which it is often compared. From time to time visitors or even staff members sample this uneaten food and find it quite good.

You have been questioned, examined, jabbed, prodded, bled, and fed. You love your family and friendly visitors, but you wish they would go home. It is an effort to entertain visitors when you are sick and unable to flee. Visitors who think they are doing you a kindness by lingering, especially with unnatural, cheery chatter, need to be shooed away. At last you can go to sleep, or so you think. Some older people still cherish the idea that they might go to a hospital to get some "rest," a sad misconception in today's hospital world. The bed feels strange. There is some constant night light, your roommate snores, or groans, or worse. The nurse pops in quietly to see if you are okay (you aren't, but why say it). The medication that has to be given every three hours wakens you twice more.

The day dawns at last; new hope arises. More consultations and tests, and finally a diagnosis is achieved and a plan of action proposed. The suspense of waiting makes for anxiety and apprehension. At this time a good nurse, social worker, chaplain, or thoughtful doctor is a godsend, because explanation and full disclosure are essential. If surgery is planned, the thought of imminent action to end your troubles is a comfort as well as a worry.

If your small child is the patient, you will probably not be permitted to remain by the bedside. This is hard for the child and for parents. Some hospitals are more humane and liberal than others about having a parent around all the time. On the other hand, if every child's parent were present all the time, the result would be an unmanageable chaos.

If you are a new mother who has spent hours in labor, the harrowing experience is soon succeeded, but not always, by pride and joy. However, in a hospital everyone seems to forget how exhausting this experience can be—how tired you feel, how fragile your emotions are, how much you need support of all kinds. Sending new mothers home the next day saves the hospital money, but it does not make them whole, or even capable of managing their lives alone. Prenatal classes and readings, with full participation by the father, have improved things a lot, by suggesting to the mother- and father-to-be what to expect and how to cope. Friendly, frequent follow-up by birthing nurses, even if only by telephone, can and often does make life a lot easier. Ideally, the patient and her family are given the telephone number of a birthing nurse and encouraged to call at any time for advice. The money saved to the health-care system through early discharge is of no use if prenatal and postnatal care are insufficient. Activist women have helped to bring about many humane changes. There is a large emotional as well as financial cost if a recently discharged mother or baby must be readmitted. Many states have considered, and some have already passed, legislation mandating a slightly longer stay after delivery.

Hospitalization for Surgery

Under managed care, patients who need surgery are referred by their primary-care doctor to a surgeon who is on an approved panel. It is not likely that patients can make an informed assessment of the surgeons available and choose a specific one, but, on the other hand, the quality of surgical care, irrespective of personal preference, will be good.

Under managed care, surgery is for the most part carried out by well-qualified surgeons whose work is scrutinized for outcomes and the number of complications, as compared to a standard norm. This is good news for patients. Managed-care surgeons are assured of sufficient work and adequate support, but they may no longer be as well paid, nor as free to be fully in command of the patient's case. The surgeon must be a member of the hospital staff with full operating privileges and be one of your health plan's approved providers. More than ever they are forced to be team players. As has been mentioned before, your surgeon is not apt to become very involved with your daily care. Another doctor will take over these tasks.

Hospitalization for Cancer

In 1994 1,170,000 new cases of cancer of all types were reported, resulting in a tremendous number of hospitalizations. No two cancers are alike, so hospitalization may fill several roles in the care of the cancer patient. Skin cancers, for example, do not require hospital admissions in most cases, unless wide excision means removing so much skin that it is necessary to do grafting. Hospital treatment of cancer involves surgical removal of the growth when possible, radiation and chemotherapy, or any combination of these three procedures.

Hospitals, all but the smallest, are required by the JCAHCO to keep a Cancer Registry. The American Cancer Society and other organizations use this information to predict trends in morbidity (disability) and mortality, and to assess the effectiveness of various types of treatment. Large numbers of patients are needed to provide valid statistics; patients are not recorded by name outside the hospital, to protect their privacy. There is also a tumor board of the staff members, which regularly reviews diagnoses, treatments, and outcomes, both good and bad, reporting these to a number of organizations and government agencies. Complex cases and ones that require extraordinary techniques such as bone marrow or organ transplants are best sent to specialized centers. Here again, you, the patient, may need to be farther from home and your family doctor, so your care may become fragmented.

In cancer hospitals, team conferences decide on each patient's treatment plan, to ensure that the treatments are coordinated. The oncologists (cancer specialists), surgeons, radiation experts, nursing service, and pharmacists agree on a plan. One specific doctor may or may not act as the chief, or primary provider, to communicate with the family. The great cancer hospitals of this country are increasingly aware of the human needs of their patients and have on their staffs specialists in pain control, social services, psychiatry, and ethics. These are vital services, but their cost-effectiveness is hard to prove, and we can only hope that the money people will take a broad view and preserve these humane services.

If you have the misfortune to be beyond help from the specialized services of the major cancer hospitals, you may be better off at home under hospice care, or in your small, local hospital where you can still see an oncologist (cancer specialist) if your family doctor thinks it advisable. In later stages of the disease, pain can almost always be controlled, even at home, by the administration of highly effective medications; the special art and science of pain control have reached higher levels in recent years. Effective medicines, and ingenious new ways of delivering pain relief, are available. There is no excuse for withholding medicine from a person in pain. No one in my experience has ever become addicted to pain-relieving medicines when they are used strictly for the relief of pain, no matter how large the dose or how long the duration of the pain. Family members need to ask questions and find out what steps to take.

The hospice movement is proving invaluable in the care of patients with advanced cancer. The hospice movement, which is nonprofit and staffed largely by volunteers, is deservedly growing rapidly. To be eligible for hospice care patients need to be thoroughly evaluated, and a fatal outcome needs to be clearly established. At that point comfort, relief of pain, and spiritual solace are established as the goals. Hospice care is usually reimbursed, at least in part, by insurers: Medicare, Medicaid, the Blues, and many managed-care plans. One criterion for eligibility is that the life expectation of the patient does not exceed six months in most cases. The patient's physicians must give a complete evaluation and prognosis, in requesting hospice care. The patient may be either at home or in a special hospice facility. The atmosphere is one of affection and caring, where appropriate pain-relieving medications are freely available.

Hospitalization for Heart Disease

Failure of the heart to be able to pump adequate amounts of blood—congestive heart failure—is the leading cause of death in this country. All general physicians are familiar with the principles of treatment for nonhospitalized patients (digitalis, ACE inhibitors, anticoagulants, diuretics, anti-arrhythmics, oxygen at times, and dietary restriction) so that hospitalization is reserved for those who, despite all measures, are getting worse. At this point a cardiologist's advice is needed (if one has not already been consulted). The justification for hospitalization is that the hospital can supply twenty-four-hour nursing, oxygen, monitoring, and surgical intervention, which is not always necessary or effective. Heart attack, the common term for coronary thrombosis, myocardial infarction, or coronary occlusion, calls for immediate hospitalization not only for confirmation of the diagnosis, which is not always apparent, but especially so that caregivers can provide the many forms of intervention now available that can limit damage and increase chances of survival. In 1995 some 7.2 million Americans were recorded as having coronary artery disease. Most of these people underwent echocardiography (ultrasound) or the expensive procedure of cardiac catheterization. There were, among this group, between 300,000 and 500,000 coronary bypass open-heart surgery procedures, at a cost of $12,000–$15,000 per procedure.

If heart disease is of particular concern for you, picking your hospital is crucial. You need to know whether there is a coronary or cardiac intensive-care unit. Are there trained cardiac-care nurses around the clock? Is there a full-time trained physician available? Can open-heart surgery, if necessary, be carried out on short notice? Rehabilitation after major cardiac surgery is a very important step in recovery. The patient and the family need information and detailed instructions on diet, exercise, sexual activity, signs of when to call for help, and above all a constantly available source of advice. Does your plan meet all of these needs? If none of these options are available, what arrangements can be made for transfer, and what are the capabilities of the next hospital and its staff? You must balance the time involved in such a transfer against the possible risks and benefits—not an easy decision.

As a heart patient you may also like to know, if possible, the attitude of the attending physician and hospital administration toward managing terminal illness. Do they honor a living will, or a health-care proxy, made out by the patient? What is their policy on DNR (do not resuscitate) orders? Families are not always in agreement about the management of terminal illness despite the previously stated wishes of the patient. I have been in the middle of such intrafamily struggles on many occasions.

The advantage of a health-care proxy is that at a time when the patient is dangerously ill, and unable to make life and death decisions, close relatives are understandably upset and highly emotional about the prospect of losing a loved one. Whereas the designated holder of the proxy is representing the patient's own wishes. The family naturally may want the patient to cling to life because they cannot face the loss.

A living will is not always respected. It may not be prominently displayed with the patient's medical record, or its existence may not even be known to the hospital staff or family doctor. Hospital policy or practices unfortunately sometimes ignore the living will.

Hospitalization for Stroke

Clots in brain arteries or hemorrhages into the brain substance produce "stroke." A stroke involves, depending on the size and location, loss of consciousness, paralysis, loss of speech, loss of all or part of vision, loss of control of bladder or bowels, or merely a temporary loss of one of these functions. Here the hospital can supply the services previously listed, such as tube feeding, skin care, catheterization, oxygen, anticoagulants, and other special treatments. Prompt early treatment can be crucially important in limiting damage. Diagnosis needs to be as rapid and precise as possible, and doctors need to lay out all the facts so that patients and family members can decide on a course of action. For example, anticoagulant drugs can prevent further clots forming, which could arrive in the brain from the heart, but anticoagulants may make a hemorrhage more severe and continuous. It is obviously not easy to make these critical decisions in a hurry, and it is equally stressful to the attending physicians and to the family.

An unconscious patient needs intensive nursing care: breathing, bladder function, bowels, bedsores, all need intervention. This is expensive care; under present circumstances, hospitals want to move such patients to a nursing home, rehabilitation center, hospice facility, or even home, as soon as possible. The patient's (previously written) living will or health-care proxy is a useful guide here.

Planning for discharge or transfer from the hospital begins as soon as possible after admission. The doctor in charge and the nurse discuss plans with the patient and family, ideally every day. A hospital cannot physically remove an unwilling patient, but can and should state the limit of time after which the patient and the patient's family will be responsible for all hospital charges. The family is ideally, but not always, urged and entitled to participate in discharge planning.

Almost no health plans (probably none) distinguish between coverage for illnesses that are not life-threatening and those that are potentially lethal. The length of hospital stay and the utilization of expensive and unusual treatments may be restricted regardless of the severity of the illness. Here the potential patient needs to be informed of the details of coverage. Since most of us act as if we were immortal and avoid reading the small print concerning coverage of fatal illnesses we do not like to think of having, unpleasant surprises can occur. As a loved one lies apparently terminally ill, the family often wants consultation with a famous specialist or even transfer to a well-known center, such as the Mayo Clinic, or some other famous teaching hospital. You need to know your hospital's policy in such cases, and who will pay for the care. For instance, can the family, working with the family doctor, arrive at a fair and humane plan of action, when the patient has deteriorated to a vegetative state, incapable of any voluntary action and unlikely ever to improve?

At such times the family is subjected to severe stress, physical, social, and financial. It is in such cases that heroines and heroes are separated from the rest, who want no part in further caring. Some will sacrifice their own comfort, money, and time to attend to the incapacitated and unresponsive family member for a long time. But I have seen others not only walk away, refusing to take responsibility, but perhaps through guilt or shame, blame the caretaking member for not doing more, thus rationalizing their own indifference.

For the most part, families do take care of their incapacitated members, as well as they are able. Sometimes there are no other family members, either at home or even at a great distance. Cultural patterns vary. Many families are truly extended, so there are more people to help share the burdens. Social welfare agencies, church organizations, and sometimes labor unions in most parts of this country are helpful resources of which you should become aware.

7

Emergency!

*Great emergencies and crises show us how much greater
our vital resources are than we had supposed.*

WILLIAM JAMES

Emergencies are inevitable; they are a part of life and come without
warning. Every person, particularly the head of a family, must plan
for the possibility of health-care emergencies. This involves knowing what services and facilities are available in your district, what is
sanctioned by your insurance plan, and as much as possible, what
the caliber is of your local emergency facility and the doctors and
nurses who staff it. As always, advance planning based on a maximum amount of reliable information is not only very important, but
wonderfully calming at a time of crisis.

Pain, anxiety, and fear carry with them a great sense of urgency.
People arriving at an emergency room only to be confronted by extensive paperwork and long periods of waiting in a backed-up line
can become impatient and angry, even irrational. There are reasons
for the paperwork and for the delays. It would be reassuring if we
knew how to define a real emergency, but this is not always possible.

Knowing what to expect of your local emergency room and how best to proceed in the event of an emergency are goals you *can* achieve.

Who Visits the Emergency Room?

The largest number of nonemergency patients who fill emergency rooms do so because they have no personal doctor, or primary-care physician, or cannot or do not even try to reach their primary-care physician. They know they cannot legally be turned away. The Health Care Financing Administration (HCFA) has a program entitled "Emergency Aid to Elderly, Disabled, and Children." In most states this program automatically entitles these people to emergency care that will be reimbursed by the government. Medicaid patients, that is, those whose income is below the poverty line, and whose medical care is thereby covered by federal and state governments, form a disproportionately large number of the emergency-room visitors since many do not have primary-care physicians. In many states physicians will not accept patients with Medicaid, so they go to an emergency room for all of their needs. However, in several states, physicians and hospitals may lose their licenses if they refuse Medicaid patients, despite the mountains of paperwork and the unsatisfactory payment mechanisms.

The triage process results in patients being seen in the order of severity and urgency of their illness or injury. An inevitable consequence is that those less seriously ill or injured must wait, often for hours, before seeing a doctor. The only remedy for the delay is to reach your primary-care doctor by telephone and arrange to be seen soon, either by him or her, or by the specialist he or she may designate. This process, though tedious, will be quicker than waiting in the emergency room.

Police and fire departments automatically take sick or injured people to the nearest emergency room, because they have neither the time nor the capability to make judgments on the injured under their care. Others who go to the emergency room, whether they are seriously injured or not, go for forensic reasons, that is, to establish claims associated with assault, auto accident, rape, or to establish a claim as a victim of an industrial accident. For victims of assault, police need to cooperate with caregivers to establish careful documentation of the circumstances and of the injury. The presence of police in the emergency room is unsettling to one and all. Emergency rooms, particularly in inner cities, also have a steady stream of victims of alcohol and drug overdose. All too often the victim is brought in, unconscious and alone, by police, so the staff has no information about the cause. These life-threatening situations tax the diagnostic and therapeutic skills of the emergency-room staff, as usually there is no history of previous illness and the doctor doesn't know what the offending substance is. Family and friends, if present, may be motivated to conceal the truth about drug use.

Finally, there are victims of natural catastrophes, such as fires, earthquakes, floods, and tornados. These are all people who are expected to and should go to the emergency room. For the rest of the people with ailments such as stomachache, back pain, fever, cough, or vomiting, going to the emergency room should be a judgment made based on sound decision making.

Exploring Your Local Emergency Room

First of all you'll want to research the emergency services available in your immediate community. The emergency room, sometimes known as an emergency ward, is usually attached to a general hospital, although there are some freestanding emergency centers run either by the municipalities, local hospitals, or by for-profit drop-in centers. The hospital emergency room may be run by the hospital staff, but commonly it is operated under contract by a team of emergency specialists, working either for a nonprofit or a for-profit corporation. Such arrangements may be a good thing, as there are many teams of well-trained emergency specialists who do nothing but that kind of work and are experts. In smaller community hospitals, very often the physician on duty is one of the regular hospital staff serving in a rotation. That physician may or may not have had specialized emergency training.

As soon as you determine the location of emergency facilities near you, and those that fit in with your health-care plan, you should visit the facility if possible and get as much information, preferably in writing, if available, about it. Among the factors you should look at are the size of the facility and the number of patients the facility can deal with within a twenty-four-hour period. It is a good idea to find out who runs the emergency facility. Is the equipment complete and up-to-date? Is the emergency room subject to a periodic inspection by the local or state board of health? Has this emergency service met the standards and certification of the Joint Commission on Accreditation of Health Care Organizations (JCAHCO)? Is there a blood bank available? Is there twenty-four-hour staffing by a registered nurse? By an M.D.? If not, is there an M.D. immediately available? On a more detailed level you should ask about the twenty-four-hour availability of anesthesia, general surgeons, an operating-room team, and specialists such as ophthalmologists and orthopedists.

Finally, you should try to find out if there is an urgent-care or walk-in facility available for referral by the emergency-room staff, so that people without life-threatening emergencies can be seen with reasonable promptness, thereby freeing up the emergency room for its proper function.

What Is an Emergency?

You may feel more at ease about using emergency facilities if you feel confident about your ability to judge whether a health problem constitutes an emergency. We might roughly classify emergencies as certain, probable, possible, or nonemergency. This classification is unofficial and not to be used as an absolute guideline.

CERTAIN EMERGENCY SITUATIONS

In the certain group are some situations that demand prompt action. Some of the principal ones are sudden onset of shortness of breath, particularly associated with blueness of the lips; irregular breathing; and a variable degree of loss of consciousness. Of course, if the patient is a person known to have heart or lung disease, the first step should be to call the specialist who knows the patient's situation so that the doctor can consult with the emergency-room staff.

Another symptom requiring urgent attention is loss of consciousness for no apparent reason. In the case of a person who is known to be prone to fainting spells, prompt recovery may permit the observers to wait and see if the person is completely recovered before contacting the primary-care physician, if possible, before proceeding to an emergency room. If the person is not prone to fainting, the obvious first diagnosis to be considered is stroke, the third most common cause for hospitalization of people forty-five or older. If a shaking convulsion precedes the loss of consciousness, inquire as soon as possible if the person is known to have epilepsy. Diabetic patients who use insulin sometimes lose consciousness from taking a dose too large under the circumstances. Knowing that the person is a diabetic is, of course, helpful. The patient may be wearing a Medic Alert wrist band that bears this or other crucial information. Increasing weakness or drowsiness preceding loss of consciousness in a person known to have diabetes is a sign that prompt treatment is vital.

A true emergency exists when there is severe pain of rapid onset anywhere in the body—chest, abdomen, head, or extremities. Here it is essential to know the person's past and recent medical history. Not all coronary heart attacks, for example, have classical symptoms of severe pain under the breastbone accompanied by weakness and profuse sweating. Often there is no warning. Recent studies have shown that many coronary occlusions produce no symptoms—evidently the brain suppresses the message. It has been known for many years that autopsies often show signs of old or recent coronary attacks in people with no such past history. One patient of mine had two major coronary attacks without pain. In the first one, he merely recalled having a profound sweat; months later a routine cardiogram revealed the damage. In his final attack, he had no pain. He merely turned to his wife and said quietly, "Mummy, I'm dying," and promptly did so. His brain at some level was aware of what was happening.

Take very seriously any sudden changes in behavior or level of consciousness, or sudden and extreme mood changes. Here the patient's primary-care doctor or close family members may be able to supply information that can help the emergency-room staff to seek out sudden psychoses, intoxication of various sorts, vascular accidents, such as strokes or behavioral changes brought about by acute infection, overdose of insulin, or heart failure. If the victim is a stranger, it is wise to look for a bracelet or neck pendant with medical information. Diabetic patients who take insulin may get an excessively low blood sugar at times for various reasons. The hypoglycemia can produce changes in behavior, as well as sweating and dizziness before unconsciousness. Sometimes people are slow to realize that their friend or loved one does not seem to be able to speak or move as usual. Such symptoms most commonly are caused by a stroke, but insulin-induced low blood sugar can cause this picture. Drunkenness is commonly erroneously diagnosed under these circumstances.

Not everyone recognizes the signs of serious intoxication, which may not be obvious to a casual or excited observer. Staggering gait, loss of balance, slurred speech, unusual or inappropriate apathy, excitement, or sudden aggressiveness are the commoner classical signs of intoxication of various sorts. Vomiting, with or without loss of control of bladder or bowels should also raise suspicion of intoxication. Best of all, knowledge of the patient's habits and recent activity is important information leading to the correct diagnosis. Remember that the offending substance, be it alcohol, cocaine, heroin, speed, or LSD, may have been taken very shortly before a patient was transported to the emergency room, and that further absorption and intoxication will continue to proceed until some intervention is begun. Immediate detoxification may even be life-saving. I recall one instance where a teenager went uninvited to a college dormitory room where there was a party. Challenged to "chug-a-lug," she drank a whole bottle of bourbon whiskey and left the party promptly on her own volition. Shortly afterward she was found unconscious under a bush by a college proctor, who happened to be a medical student. His prompt action in getting her to an emergency room undoubtedly saved her life.

The victim of assault always needs immediate attention. No matter if the injuries seem trivial at the time, a complete history and physical examination of the patient is a must. Very often the victim has reasons to resist examination such as fear, shame, or concealment of involvement in criminal activity. This may lead the victim to minimize the injury. Quite often injured people who appear to have sustained only a superficial gunshot wound, when carefully examined, are found to have other bullet or stab wounds that were not spoken of at first. The police must always be notified.

A suicide attempt is a dangerous emergency. This must be taken seriously, very seriously indeed. Not only are all resuscitative measures called for, but follow-up is all important. Second attempts at suicide within twenty-four or forty-eight hours of the first attempt are extremely common, so close observation is essential. Emergency-room staff will need to identify a responsible person who will continue this surveillance for days or even weeks. It is extremely important to have a social worker or psychotherapist assigned to the case before the patient leaves the emergency room.

Sexual abuse, even probable or possible abuse, is a true emergency. A person may conceal the damage because of fear or shame. Here is an occasion when openness, accurate observation, and truthfulness are essential. The victim should be carefully examined for evidence of injury, and the police should be informed for follow-up. The victim's needs are far more important than protection of an alleged perpetrator's reputation. Special counseling should begin at once, because covering up or trivializing sexual abuse always brings lifelong fears, anxiety, and anger.

Look out for shaking chills and high fever. Alternating sweats, chills, and prostration are also true emergencies as they may represent pneumonia, overwhelming urinary tract infection, streptococcal infection (as in the toxic shock syndrome), septicemia (blood poisoning), or even the onset of such diseases as meningitis, malaria, typhoid, and typhus. Again, it is assumed that the patient will try to reach a primary-care doctor before going to the emergency room.

Immediately after a burn from fire or boiling water, the damage may not look serious. But burns that involve blistering and loss of skin are true emergencies and should be treated as such. Home remedies usually do more harm than good.

An injury from smoke inhalation, usually at the scene of a fire, can produce serious damage to the lungs and interference with oxygenation of the brain. Smoke inhalation is potentially fatal. In the great Coconut Grove Nightclub fire in Boston in 1942, of the hundreds of serious and fatal injuries, more harm was done by smoke inhalation than by skin burns. Sometimes fire victims require further specialized treatment and need to be transported by air to one of the few facilities that has high-pressure oxygen breathing equipment (hyperbaric chambers). Such treatments must begin as soon as possible.

Profound weakness and helplessness may be a sign of shock. This is a medical term that describes the symptoms produced by a drop in blood pressure and failure of circulation. Shock may be brought on by injury, internal bleeding, poisoning, severe burns, overwhelming infection, or other causes. The person in shock may be unconscious or intermittently conscious, perhaps confused, pale, and sweating with a very weak, rapid pulse. Prompt treatment of shock is life-saving.

In assessing a severe sprain or fracture, it is not always possible to tell at the scene the exact nature of the injury. People with injuries to the hip, neck, and back should be transported only by a trained emergency crew, such as those attached to most fire and/or police departments. Do not try to move the injured person by yourself. Most particularly do not move a person who complains of back or neck pain.

A painless but nevertheless potentially very serious symptom is a sudden loss of vision. There are various causes, all serious, including obstruction in an artery to the brain or in the eye itself, detachment of the retina, or in rare instances poisoning from drinking wood (methyl) alcohol. It is critically important to deal with this promptly as some conditions such as retinal detachment or closure of a small artery behind the eye can produce permanent blindness unless promptly treated.

A severe headache associated with stiff neck, with or without fever, may indicate hemorrhage, undetected brain injury, or meningitis. In infants particularly, violent vomiting (projectile vomiting) is a serious sign, as it may represent increased intracranial pressure.

Inability to urinate is most commonly seen in cases of enlargement of the prostate in older men. After several hours of trying unsuccessfully to urinate, there is not only great pain, but damage to the kidneys from back pressure. The bladder must be emptied promptly. It usually is relieved for the time being by catheterization of the bladder. Failure to follow up and have definitive treatment of the cause of the obstruction will only result in further attacks.

Delirium tremens, which generally follows withdrawal from a

long spell of intoxication, usually with alcohol, is sometimes referred to as if it were a joke, but it is indeed a life-threatening condition and may last for many days. The proper treatment in an emergency room may be life-saving.

Typically, the person with DTs, as the condition is called, is confused, excited, speaking irrationally, sometimes displaying active hallucinations and delusions, with shaking hands and head.

PROBABLE EMERGENCY CONDITIONS

There comes next a class of health situations that are not usually quite as urgent. We might call these probable emergencies. This is a varied group of ailments that call for prompt but not immediate attention and should, if possible, be dealt with *outside* of the emergency room. These include gradual loss of vision or hearing, progressive impairment of movement of the arms and legs, difficulty speaking, or diminished level of awareness. These conditions may probably require careful examination by the primary-care doctor or a neurologist. Continuing confusion, mood change, delusions, and hallucinations may indicate psychosis such as schizophrenia or intoxication, but to examine the patient properly will require more time and detail than can be delivered in the emergency room. Since they are not life-threatening conditions, little harm is done if the patient waits to be seen by the appropriate physicians.

Everyone has at some time experienced severe vomiting and diarrhea. Making a judgment about the potential dangerousness of the condition may be very difficult. The common gastroenteritis, which may be a result of food poisoning or more commonly a germ transmitted through the air from person to person, certainly makes the patient feel and look very ill, but it is almost always self-limited. A telephone call to someone who was at the same meeting or ate the same meal, or was at the same school, can give valuable information about the cause and likely outcome. The causes of epidemics of vomiting and diarrhea are only identified in about 20 percent of the cases even by the experts of the Centers for Disease Control in Atlanta. Local health departments have even less success in identifying causes.

It is reasonable, and in fact desirable, to keep the sick person, be it child or adult, at home for as long as possible. The exception to this rule is in the case of infants, who can become severely dehydrated, with potentially serious consequences, after only a few hours of vomiting and diarrhea and will need intravenous replacement. People who have severe, insulin-dependent diabetes are also at risk.

Anyone who experiences vomiting and diarrhea persisting for over twenty-four hours should seek medical attention. This does not mean rushing to the emergency room, but preferably you should get in touch with your primary-care provider. It is a good idea to try simple remedies at first.

Severe migraine headache is not life-threatening, but sometimes it may best be referred to an emergency room because of the availability of an injectable substance (sumatriptan) that may bring dramatic relief. In a typical severe migraine attack, the sufferer wants to be alone, in a completely quiet, dark room and may prefer to avoid going to the hospital.

Acute earache in children is best dealt with by the pediatrician, and not in the emergency room. Untreated middle-ear infections are not only extremely painful but can, on occasion, lead to deafness.

Asthma is one of the most common conditions seen in all emergency facilities and, for reasons not altogether clear, such cases are increasing in frequency, especially among minority children. Severe attacks can be life-threatening. Simply giving the patient medicine to relieve the spasm and ease the breathing and then discharging him or her from the emergency room more often than not results in a prompt return to the emergency room within twenty-four hours. Asthma is better treated over a period of time by a primary-care doctor who is familiar with the causes of the attacks and the behavior of the patient. An asthma patient who has used the previously prescribed medicine as directed (usually a spray) and who is still very short of breath is at risk and needs prompt care. Treatment in the emergency room by appropriate bronchodilator or steroid spray, or both, is best followed by an observation period in a non-emergency area, since acute attacks often recur within a short time.

Possible Emergency Situations

Less serious are what we might call possible emergencies. Rapid weight gain may indicate accumulation of fluid in the heart, or kidney failure, but it is not an immediate emergency. Generalized muscular weakness or spells of drowsiness occurring over a period of days or weeks need prompt but not immediate attention.

Frequent urination may represent impending prostatic obstruction in men or urinary-tract infection in either sex, or it may be the first sign of diabetes. In either case such complaints are best dealt with in the doctor's office. A simple urine test very often will determine the cause, and the symptoms usually will respond to simple antibiotic or other appropriate treatment.

Now you should have a rough idea when to use and when to avoid the emergency room. It is well to discuss with your doctor, or the case manager in your health-care plan, nonurgent but same-day services available to you, where your waiting period may be shorter and you may have more time with the doctor and nurse.

Going to the Emergency Room

Having decided that an emergency-room visit is necessary, there are ways to proceed. First of all, bring with you, if you have them available, your immunization records, and particularly in the case of injuries, the date of your last tetanus booster. Put in writing the significant parts of your medical history and of the present illness. Most important, never forget to take with you your insurance card and all the medications you are taking. The person receiving you and doing the triaging will then be in a position to deal with your problem more promptly.

Be sure you are going to the right emergency room. That is, one approved by your plan and one that you have determined in advance has the capabilities already mentioned. Call ahead to the emergency room if you possibly can, or have someone do it for you. Be sure that someone calls your primary-care physician so that he or she can coordinate with the emergency-room staff and perhaps save you a good deal of time. Your primary-care physician under most plans must approve this emergency-room visit in order to ensure coverage by your health plan.

If you are alone, this may be the time, if you are ambulatory, to take a taxi, since your injury or illness may make driving dangerous, and parking near emergency rooms is invariably very difficult. You can also call your health plan to find out under what circumstances ambulance services are available and will be paid for. Be sure that the ambulance that you call will take you to the emergency room you want. Simply dialing 911 without asking some questions may result in being taken to the wrong facility. Some ambulance services have arrangements with certain emergency facilities to deliver patients to them. Although this may be an unethical practice, unfortunately it does occur. Another barrier is that sometimes municipal ambulances run by towns or police or fire departments may be, by regulation, forbidden to take patients to any hospital other than the nearest local hospital. Automobile-accident victims brought in by the police, particularly if unconscious, sometimes end up in the wrong emergency room. To get transferred to another facility is usually very difficult and may not be a wise move, depending on the victim's condition.

In all systems there is generally a clerk who first receives people coming in and tries to get as much relevant detail as possible in order to facilitate treatment. The next person is usually a nurse whose function is known as triage. "Triage" is a French military term indicating the sorting out of those who are beyond help from those who genuinely need prompt attention for life-threatening illnesses or injuries and from those who have needs that, although distressing to them, are not as urgent. To the patient or victim, his or her own needs, of course, are the most important, and to be told to wait while a more recent arrival is attended to understandably causes dissatisfaction. In a perfect world everyone would have a primary-care doctor who could be reached by telephone all day, every day, and who would decide whether the ailment warranted an immediate visit to the emergency room, but this is obviously impossible. If such an ideal situation existed, no emergency room would be as crowded nor would delays be as long as they are at present.

When you are finally ushered into an examining room and have the attention of the nurse or doctor, try to tell your medical story of symptoms in sequence. Do not diagnose yourself, but try to give an objective description of what you are experiencing. Be sure to tell caregivers about any known allergies or intolerance to any medication. If you, or the person you are transporting, has been a victim of violence, sexual abuse, or any sort of family struggle, this is not the time to hide a guilty secret; you need to be frank and open. There are in many jurisdictions laws mandating disclosure of such abuse, and concealment of this information by any person with such knowledge is a felony.

The details of your visit to the emergency room are recorded as required by the JCAHCO. Your primary-care doctor can obtain a copy of the record, and you should have one also. You need to know the diagnosis, the treatment given, and any arrangements for follow-up. You will not be given more than one or two days of medication.

You and your own doctor need to discuss this as soon as possible. Of course, your visit may necessitate hospitalization. If so, be sure that your doctor and your insurance plan are aware of your admission. I'm sorry to say that these essential communications do not always take place.

Again, I must emphasize that knowing yourself, your own needs and weaknesses, or those of your family members, combined with knowing what health-care facilities are available to you, leads to a sense of self-confidence and makes it easier for you to plan how to proceed in the event of an emergency. Only you can decide whether it is worse to be careless of health or excessively concerned.

8

Alternative Medicine

Skepticism is the highest of duties,
blind faith the one unpardonable sin.

Thomas Henry Huxley

Books, magazine stories, and television dramas almost always depict
M.D.'s, R.N.'s and others working in emergency rooms and hospital
operating rooms. Most of the public debate over health-care reform
and financing relates to the established medical system. There are
no dramas on TV having to do with life in the office of a chiropractor or acupuncturist. Meditation and yoga may make dull fare for
TV, yet a huge number of Americans are turning away from conventional medical care to try other approaches. Many of these alternative pathways have roots that antedate modern establishment
medicine by centuries. Entire civilizations in the East, in Africa,
and in America use and have faith in forms of treatment that are
effective in ways that American medicine ignores, to its own detriment. Thousands of practitioners study and believe in a variety of
approaches and they have millions of satisfied patients.

In a landmark article in 1993 in the *New England Journal of Med-*

icine, Dr. David M. Eisenberg and his colleagues described the nature and extensiveness of "unconventional medicine in the United States." They pointed out that there are two "tracks" for those seeking primary care. The first, termed "scientific" medicine, is of the familiar, well-described, heavily regulated, and heavily financed variety. The other track is "alternative" or "unconventional" care and includes a wide range of belief systems and a wide range of organizations, largely not subject to government supervision or regulation, although there are licensing standards in some states as well as accrediting organizations.

Eisenberg and his colleagues pointed out that the frequency of the use of unconventional therapy in the United States is far higher than had been previously reported. One-third of the 1,539 adults he interviewed had used at least one unconventional therapy in the last year, and about one in nine had gone repeatedly to an alternative-care provider, for an average of nineteen visits, with an average charge of $27.60 a visit. Over half of all this money was paid out of pocket by the patients. Those going to unconventional therapy for the most part had also gone to a medical doctor first and usually did not tell their own doctor of the other visits. The total spent on unconventional therapy out of pocket, some $10.3 billion in 1993, is enormous and should be considered in any revision of our health-care payment system. The Eisenberg team calculated that in one year there are about 425 million visits to providers of nonconventional therapy.

Modern "scientific" medicine, sometimes referred to as "allopathic medicine," traditionally holds that the cause of an ailment should be objectively identified and the treatment based on reasoning from analysis of established facts. Medical progress, however, has often been based on false assumptions and has proceeded by trial and error. M.D.'s who are not aware of medical history may assume that the causes of certain illnesses have been proven, and that treatments are effective because the link between the therapy and improved health can be established logically. But some ailments remain chronic and intractable. For instance, sufferers from chronic back pain are often disappointed on both counts, as neither cause nor cure can be predicted. Instead the treatment that relieves the pain is the one in which patients put credence. When their regular health-care system does not and cannot provide help, it is not to be wondered at that they look elsewhere, despite costs or warnings. People need hope; that is what they so often find in alternative health care.

Unfortunately, there has been little rigorous objective testing, using commonly accepted scientific standards, of the effectiveness or the safety of the innumerable methods or substances involved in these, for the most part, unregulated treatments. Under congressional mandate, the National Institutes of Health established in 1992 a division to study alternative treatments. Probably regulation by the Food and Drug Administration will follow as soon as there are data on which to base guidelines and rules. There are also centers for studies of alternative medicine at, among others, Columbia College of Physicians and Surgeons, Harvard Medical School, Temple University, and the Universities of Miami and Maryland.

Dr. Andrew Weil has for years been studying and promoting natural healing — the remarkable powers often seen when mind and body are given the opportunity and support for healing themselves. He writes knowledgeably about alternative therapies as well as their underlying philosophies. His books are well worth reading by anyone interested in the forces governing health and illness. His background and training in the study of science in its broadest sense are impressive, and his credentials in the medical academic community are impeccable. He cannot be accused of being ignorant of rigorous scientific research methods. Respected academic physicians with the training and stature of Drs. Weil, Eisenberg, and others have started a wave of fresh thinking and investigation.

Opponents of alternative medicine say that these treatments are based on faulty science, or no science. For that matter, the same finger could be pointed at the dominant "scientific" medicine. We need only recall that the Nobel laureate, Dr. Linus Pauling's advocacy of high daily doses of vitamin C, derided by most medical scientists at the time, seems now, at least in part, to have been justified. To give another example, the early opposition to routine radical surgery for all breast cancers, the gold standard from 1900 to the 1970s, seems now to be correct. Many doctors now practicing can recall when anything short of radical mastectomy was considered gross malpractice. They have changed their tune. The study of science suggests the need for humility. The eminent mathematician-philosopher Alfred North Whitehead once referred to "misplaced scientific precision." Many scientists today seem so preoccupied by statistical methodology that common sense may suffer. As Dr. Thomas L. Delbanco asks: "How many approaches to multiple regression now exist? Which statistical inference is right for the latest set of data? In 1994 is butter or margarine safer?" After other examples he continues, "So even at a time of rich scientific endeavor and discovery, patients turn to plants or homeopathic distillates and announce, I would rather swallow this! It's pure, it's safe, it's magic, and it will help me face the world." Magic is what every sufferer seeks from any healing system, conventional or otherwise.

The concerned citizen judges the effectiveness of, for example, herbal therapy or of acupuncture in two ways—by anecdote and by the results of controlled trials. So far there have been almost no controlled trials for most alternative therapies, so anecdote must remain the chief source of information. Anecdote tells of the wonderful outcome for one person of one treatment at one time, but it cannot predict outcomes for many other people being treated for other ailments at other times. There are very few anecdotes of treatment failures, and there are more believers than doubters in, for example, acupuncture and homeopathy.

Controlled trials are expensive and time-consuming. Such trials should be funded by our government, as they have been to some extent in Germany. Pharmaceutical manufacturers, sensing the possibility of large profits, have showed some interest in alternative medications and treatments, but cannot be expected to provide comprehensive and disinterested evaluation. The observers must be aware of their own and others' biases. This objectivity is rare and hard to develop. We can hope and even expect that the newer approach by the NIH and medical schools will provide some useful guidelines. Inevitably there will be more legal standards, accreditation bodies, and special licensure, which will drive up costs.

The decision of whether or not to use an alternative therapy is difficult. People without health insurance often make the decision solely on financial grounds, because often herbal or homeopathic medicines, massages, or spinal adjustments may cost less than a visit to a medical doctor. In practice, this may not prove to be cost saving, because for chronic ailments some of the therapies call for commitment to a long course of treatments. This raises the question of whether in a democratic society taxpayers should pay for care or treatment they do not believe in, but that is at present only part of the ongoing large debate, political more than philosophical. The present Republican party has proposed a voucher system for health care, whereby people can be helped to pay for whatever treatments they choose. Senator Edward Kennedy, who has a long interest in universal health care, is among those who feel that such a system would lead to unequal distribution of care. As everyone's taxes go at present to support the present medical systems, some regulations must be devised to subsidize other forms of care, probably with some governmental system of evaluation of effectiveness. Claims made by both conventional medicine and some of the alternatives have sometimes been exaggerated, and a skeptical attitude is useful. For each of the flamboyant claims for various alternatives, there are also press releases promising breakthroughs issued by medical schools, hospitals, and pharmaceutical firms. In any case, people want relief of suffering and something they can believe in.

Among the many alternative therapies, the most widely used and well entrenched deserve consideration here. These descriptions are for the most part not based on my own personal experience, but represent the choices of thousands, probably millions, of Americans. I believe all approaches should be explored, and critical studies of effectiveness, financed by federal tax funds, not by interested parties, should be instituted.

Very few alternative or "unconventional" therapists adhere to a rigid, narrow approach. Acupuncturists, for example, usually prescribe herbs, diet, and massage as well. Massage therapists may also employ hydrotherapy, aromatherapy, and relaxation techniques. First there are treatments based on diets of all sorts, herbal therapy, and aromatherapy, using foods, herbs, plant and flower extracts, and essential oils. Second there are spirituality or belief-based systems, including Christian Science, Seventh-Day Adventism, yoga, transcendental meditation, and relaxation techniques. Faith in any belief system undoubtedly has beneficial effects, which are impossible to measure. Third there are treatments based on application of more or less complex theories: acupuncture, acupressure, chiropractic, homeopathy, reflexology, color therapy, and dance therapy. Fourth there are treatments employing direct physical application such as exercise, hydrotherapy, massage, and light and sound treatment.

Combinations of the above may be used in holistic medicine, naturopathy, and homeopathy. Doctors of medicine often refer their patients for massage or chiropractic treatment, sometimes concealing this practice from their colleagues. Naturopathic doctors often combine counseling, botanical medicine, diets, and homeopathy. There is a board of certification in naturopathy, and in many states a licensing board as well.

Diet, Herbal Therapy, and Aromatherapy

Looking briefly at the first category of treatments, we recognize that diets of various forms are among the most fundamental and ancient practices, often incorporated into the customs, religion, and even the laws of various civilizations. The idea that "you are what you eat" seems to have a fundamental appeal to people. When we consider the enormous variety of food substances on which people subsist on this planet, and all survive, it is difficult to imagine that there is one diet that is "right" and one that is "wrong." From earliest times warriors have consumed the brain, heart, testes, or other organs of defeated victims to gain some desired attributes, but this custom is no longer prevalent.

There are innumerable variations of the "healthy" diet. Thousands of Americans are vegetarians. Their health by all objective standards is usually excellent, and they have considerably less coronary heart disease and other signs of hardening of the arteries. Some diets are based on progressive elimination of foods that cause adverse reactions. Allergists have for years tracked down various forms of food intolerance by eliminating first one, then another item from the diet. For example, the absence of the digestive enzyme lactase, a condition known as lactose intolerance, produces indigestion and diarrhea in many people and is well known to pediatricians, who prescribe avoidance of products derived from cow's milk.

Diet therapies of all sorts have always been a preoccupation in this country. We only need to remember in the nineteenth century the flourishing of the sanatorium in Battle Creek, followed by the disciples of Dr. Kellogg, and the enduring legacy of corn flakes and related cereals. Dr. Graham, who was honored by the department of medicine at Yale for his work, was an advocate of a kind of unrefined flour, and he is still remembered for inventing the graham cracker. Along with other imports from oriental philosophy in the 1960s and 1970s, the "macrobiotic" diet had a tremendous vogue that has not yet died out. It is based on an elaborate theory of an ascending order of purity of foods. The most pure diet recommended is one that most professional nutritionists agree is grossly incomplete and inadequate. Indeed, macrobiotic diets are usually used nowadays only for short periods of time for "purging" the system of supposed impurities by confining intake to a small number of cereal grains. Low-fat diets, of course, are now the darling of the cardiovascular experts. Low-carbohydrate diets are supposed by many to reduce violent, aggressive behavior. In fact, in one notorious murder case the defense was that the perpetrator had a great sweet tooth, which produced violent aggression after the defendant gorged on candies. That type of defense is known in legal circles as the "Twinkie defense." There was even a bill introduced in the California legislature to compel a low-starch diet for all violent convicted criminals.

Seeing and hearing all of the advertisements for vitamins and megavitamins, we wonder, are they necessary? Over half of adult Americans take vitamin supplements, according to the industry. There are no figures to show that people who take vitamins are healthier than those people who don't. Vitamins are substances essential in minute quantities in the human body for regulating or participating in various important chemical or physiological functions of the body. They are present in adequate amounts in the diets of most Americans living above the poverty line. True deficiencies are very uncommon in this country, and then usually in people who have serious intestinal malfunction or who, because of alcoholism, drug abuse, or poverty eat a grossly inadequate diet. Nevertheless, it is a popular belief, reinforced by advertising, that taking vitamins can promote better health. There is no scientific evidence to support this claim, according to the National Research Council, which periodically revises the recommended daily allowances of each vitamin. Excesses of vitamins A and D can actually be harmful since they are fat soluble and can accumulate in the body and be difficult to eliminate from the system. On the other hand, recent re-ports in the press have indicated that in animal experiments the "antioxidant" vitamins A, C, and E may have some protective ac-tion against heart or blood-vessel diseases, even some cancers, and have attracted much attention. However, there are few human stud-ies or statistics to confirm these findings. At the very least it seems clear that vitamins in moderate amounts are harmless and inexpen-sive, but they are not magic bullets. It is unreasonable to escalate daily intake to levels that might possibly be harmful (megavitamins) as a trade-off to eating a balanced diet including natural, fresh foods.

Herbal medicine has a wide and enthusiastic following. Herbal medicine as it is commercially applied in this country is largely de-rived from Chinese sources and European and North American medicinal herbs. At the same time, the use of natural remedies by the natives of both North and South America has also, since time immemorial, had a large following; these are increasingly the sub-jects of study and use.There are now over 550 medicinal herbs available in the United States according to Madeline Drexler, writ-ing in the *Boston Globe Magazine*. It may be surprising to note that nearly half of all the medications listed in the *Physicians Desk Ref-erence*, the bible of prescription drugs, come from plant sources.

According to Dr. David Eisenberg, some 3 percent of people in the United States use herbal remedies of one sort or another. Indus-try sources report that the therapeutic herbal industry is growing at a rate of 15 percent annually (compared with the pharmaceutical industry's annual growth rate of 4 percent). Some of the more popu-lar herbs, and their reported effects, are ginseng (for alertness), chamomile (for its calming properties), gingerroot (for motion sick-ness), Mormon tea (for bronchospasm, as in asthma), raspberry leaf (for diarrhea), and peppermint (for gastric discomfort). It seems that everyone's grandmother or great-grandmother had a favorite tonic or remedy. The Native Americans knew of the effectiveness of teas derived from birch bark, which they used in the treatment of muscle and joint pain long before salicylates (which they contain) were synthesized and introduced as aspirin. In this country we are only beginning to categorize and fix specifications for such substances.

To date there are no studies on herbs that begin to approach the careful clinical and laboratory studies that the FDA imposes on prescription drugs. Vague claims are still permissible ("useful for rheumatic imbalances," "stimulates digestion," "helpful in cases of loss of sexual function"), but it is not permissible to make specific medicinal claims. Mark Blumenthal of the American Botanical Council in Texas informed Ms. Drexler that the German government sponsored thorough scientific monographs on 324 herbal treatments, and he notes that of these, 100 were not approved. Some of these 100 herbs not approved in Germany are widely available in stores in the United States. We may expect more reliable information from the studies proposed in this country in the near future. As for information now available, Madeline Drexler describes Michael Kassleman's *The Healing Herbs* and Varrow Tyler's *Herbs of Choice*, as reliable.

We do not know as much as we would like about some herbal remedies. In April 1996, the FDA issued a warning against the use of dietary supplements containing the stimulant ephedrine, marketed under various names, notably Herbal Ecstasy. The FDA had compiled 400 reports of side effects, including heart attacks, convulsive seizures, and psychoses. Fifteen people had died after taking these supplements. Ephedrine is a common ingredient in some nonprescription asthma medicine and is an important ingredient in the illegal drug methamphetamine or "speed." The manufacturers of herbal remedies containing ephedrine promote their products as "natural" and safe, often listing them under the plant name ephedra or the Chinese plant name ma huang. Before using ephedrine to lose weight or boost energy, the conservative person will want to wait until this country has conducted some more organized authoritative evaluations of such substances.

Since Roman times, herbal extracts of the plant known as pennyroyal have been alleged to bring about abortion. This herb is widely available over the counter in health-food stores. The effectiveness of pennyroyal in producing abortion has never been critically evaluated. Four cases of poisoning from its use, one of which was fatal, were reported in San Francisco in 1996.

Prior to 1994 there was little supervision of over-the-counter herbal remedies. However, in 1994, after an unprecedented barrage of letters and calls, Congress passed the deceptively named Dietary Supplemental Health and Education Act. This legislation relieved the manufacturers from having to demonstrate the safety of their products before marketing them. The labels on over-the-counter products should be read with care. The law now limits the claims on labels to general terms, but it does not prevent specific claims in newspaper or magazine advertisements, which sometimes promise cures of incurable conditions and offer great hopes to the uninformed. It is safer to read the label and to look up the substance in a reputable herbal book. The FDA can now only attempt to prove that these substances are unsafe after they have been placed on the market. There is, furthermore, at present no legal limit on unjustified and sweeping health claims. According to a *New York Times* article, Dr. Richard Friedman of the Cornell Medical Center called the FDA to ask this question: Suppose I wanted to sell hemlock tea, the deadly poison that Socrates drank? The FDA replied that "until the bodies piled up," hemlock tea could be freely sold.

Other groups of naturally occurring substances have been elevated to the status of healing substances. Flower remedies have a considerable following. An English physician, Dr. Edward Bach, before his death in 1936, had written extensively on the medicinal use of flowers, scents, or extracts, either inhaled or tasted, in conjunction with other therapy. Each emotion or feeling, according to Dr. Bach and his followers in the Flower Essence Society, can be helped by the appropriate flower. Today flower-remedy treatment is used not as the only treatment but in conjunction with other forms of therapy by practitioners of naturopathic and holistic medicine. Some therapies of oriental origin also involve the use of flowers in various forms.

Aromatherapy, which is akin to flower therapy, involves the use of various scents in the form of essential oils of specific plants to treat symptoms such as depression and congestion. This practice has been in existence since the civilizations of ancient Egypt. Some sixty years ago, aromatherapy was once again popularized, first in France and then throughout Western Europe and the Western Hemisphere. Every sizable American bookstore has many titles on the subject these days, often as many as fifteen or twenty of such works.

Spiritual Systems and Meditation Therapy

Advocates of spiritual or religious-based healing systems often claim partial or even total control of health and disease if followers adhere to their tenets. Christian Science, Seventh-Day Adventism, and the Unification Church of the Reverend Sun Myung Moon are three of the more prominent examples. In rural societies in this country, as well as elsewhere, many small sects and cults flourish. Some Haitians in this country still secretly practice and believe in voodoo. Spiritual beliefs do not in most cases preclude trying other methods of healing at the same time. Opposition to the compulsory immunization of children on religious grounds comes from a small but vocal minority. This stance obviously poses a problem for schools and public-health authorities; documented outbreaks of measles and poliomyelitis have occurred among many groups opposed to immunization on religious grounds.

Many years ago while practicing in a small town, I came to know socially and be friendly with a group of people who were members of a religious sect that does not believe in medicine, but solely in the healing power of faith. I must have struck some of them as being somewhat open-minded and not vehemently opposed to their sect, as are most doctors. After a while, one or two of them would telephone me occasionally for an opinion—always insisting that they did not want treatment, and requesting that I not tell anyone about the call. Finally one family asked me to call on their mother— after dark, so that no one would see a doctor's car there. The complaint was that she had for several days been having spells of sudden onset of shortness of breath, coughing, occasionally associated with sharp chest pain, and coughing up blood. She was an elderly woman who had an obvious case of thrombophlebitis of one leg (clotted veins). I did not need an X ray (which they in any case would have refused) to tell that she was having pulmonary emboli—clots breaking loose from her leg, going through the right side of the heart, and lodging in the lung. In the conventional medicine in which I had been trained, this condition constitutes a real emergency, since the emboli are often fatal. The old woman had indeed been fortunate up to that time. I felt that she needed immediate hospitalization to have the veins tied off at the groin to prevent further emboli, and that then she should be placed on anticoagulants to prevent further clotting. The family and the patient refused. They did, however, ask me to visit daily, to observe and to give my assessment of her progress. For another week or so she continued to have these episodes; then they stopped. Her leg gradually became less red and swollen. The family, of course, felt that faith and prayer had cured their mother, and I received no credit, although they thanked me for my attention and confidentiality. I pondered then, and I still do, whether faith accelerated the healing; to some extent I believe it did, although there is no way of proving it.

Two valuable lessons came from this unusual episode. I had the very rare opportunity of observing the natural course of this dangerous condition untreated, which would never have been allowed to proceed in a teaching hospital. I learned that a series of large emboli are not always fatal, and that, as so often happens, the healing powers of the body are underestimated.

Meditation as a form of gaining or maintaining health is one of the great contributions of Eastern religion and culture to Western thought. Meditation as a form of relaxation therapy is widely advocated in many of the alternative therapies. There are many followers of meditation in Ayurvedic medicine, which is a healing system originating in India, many thousands of years old. The approach is based on the belief that there are three psychophysical types of people, each requiring a different approach. This involves much meditation as well as adherence to a vegetarian diet and breathing exercises. Practitioners of Ayurvedic medicine in India undergo five years of training. Some thirty years ago there was a formal movement embracing transcendental meditation. The goals of T.M., as it is popularly called, are primarily to achieve peace of mind and a greater sense of self-awareness. Improvement of health is a secondary purpose. I have seen impressive improvements in T.M.-practicing patients with high blood pressure and anxiety conditions.

Yoga, originating in India, is a form of gaining more control of bodily processes through meditation, rigorous self-discipline, and exercise. Yoga involves sitting or taking certain bodily postures, and doing breathing exercises, often silently repeating a personal key word or phrase known as a mantra to induce a trancelike state. These exercises and the contemplation of the nature of holiness produce, according to its devotees, a serenity and detachment from bodily concerns that is satisfying. These techniques are often used to treat anxiety and depression.

Most medical education, at present, acknowledges to a greater or lesser degree the effectiveness of meditation and other relaxation techniques, such as breathing exercises, in assisting healing processes, and there is a considerable body of research demonstrating the value of such techniques in alleviating a wide variety of physical and mental disorders. Managed-care plans generally do not supply or pay for such treatment unless it is carried out by one of their physicians, who must make a definite diagnosis and adhere to strict guidelines. If you have an indemnity plan, inquire about coverage for such treatment.

Alternative Healing Systems

Many alternative treatments have grown out of larger systems of belief. For instance, acupuncture is part of Chinese medicine, while homeopathy is a system of healing that developed alongside Western medicine.

ACUPUNCTURE

Acupuncture is *one* of the "eight limbs" of Chinese medicine, which include diet, exercise, massage, herbology, and others. The treatment involves the stimulation of certain carefully designated points on the body's surface by needles or heat. According to Chinese medicine, these points lie along energy channels, also known as meridians. The acupuncturist manipulates energy flow in such a way that various organs are strengthened and physiological processes are balanced. The technique has been refined over many centuries in China and elsewhere in Asia. The cost of the average acupuncture treatment in this country is about $60. There are over ten million acupuncture treatments administered each year, and most frequently acupuncturists are asked to help patients control pain and to alleviate various ailments, including addiction. One interesting result is that the treatment is apparently successful in a high percentage of cases in helping addicts break addiction to tobacco, alcohol, or drugs.

Acupuncture has encountered, and still faces, great difficulty overcoming the skepticism of those schooled in the tenets of "scientific" medicine. There are a number of schools teaching acupuncture in the United States at this time, but acupuncturists in many states are not yet licensed to practice their specialty except in the capacity of an assistant working under the supervision of a licensed medical practitioner. Nevertheless, there are thousands of acupuncturists flourishing in many places, and they have thousands of highly satisfied clients. Most acupuncturists at this time take a holistic approach in that they take a medical history, they consider the social and psychological background of the patient, and the patient's general way of living and attitude toward life. So the acupuncture treatment is supplemented with advice on diet and living habits and may be combined with massage techniques.

The attitude of academic medicine toward acupuncture has been politely skeptical in an uninformed way. Yet more and more medical practitioners encourage their patients with intractable pain or chemotherapy-induced nausea to seek relief through acupuncture, and their physicians are gratified by the results. The use of marijuana for this same chemotherapy-induced nausea is opposed by many legal authorities, although many, perhaps a majority, of oncologists (cancer specialists) swear by its effectiveness. The resistance of the FDA to approving marijuana as a treatment is part of a long tradition of organized medicine identifying with the advocates of the "war on drugs" who see marijuana as a dangerous first step on the downward path to addiction to hard drugs. Acupuncture, I am sure, will continue to play an increased role in the management of advanced cancer. Adverse effects seem to be uncommon. Here, once again, more objective study and recommendations from the National Institutes of Health in their new explorations of alternative medicine will be helpful. Many anesthesiologists have also studied the relief of pain by acupuncture and have from time to time used these techniques.

In 1994, a group of 9,000 acupuncturists sought approval by the FDA which would entitle acupuncturists to collect from third-party insurance payers, at least for some conditions. The acupuncturists in their petition to the FDA argued that the tiny needles used in this therapy are safe and effective and should not be considered 'experimental.' This is an entirely new field for the FDA, which is now forced to make evaluations and to arrive at some sorts of decisions. This petition by the acupuncturists requested approval for five applications, namely the treatment of chronic pain, vomiting (usually following chemotherapy), alcohol and drug addiction, respiratory disorders (especially asthma), and rehabilitation for paralysis in stroke victims. A number of scientific studies were quoted by the proponents of this search for approval. Among the arguments advanced are testimonials by acupuncture patients who have had marvelous results. Enthusiasts presume that these marvelous results may be achieved for most other people, but critics demand proof, despite the testimony of five thousand years of practice.

It seems likely that within the near future acupuncture in some form will be legal and more widely accepted, more widely used, and probably more widely reimbursed by health-care insurance than at present.

The areas identified as energy pathways in acupuncture are not always stimulated by a needle. There is, in fact, a large school of treatment called *acupressure,* which involves applying manual pressure on various of the acupuncture points on the body's surface. Rhythmic pressure on these points is the essential feature of the therapy known as *shiatsu.*

HOMEOPATHY

Another large and commonly used system of treatment is known as *homeopathy*. Christian Friederich Hahnemann, the founder of homeopathy, received his M.D. in 1779 in Germany. He spent years after that studying the effects of drugs and became increasingly impressed by the harmful effects of the medications then in use. In that respect he did the medical profession and the public a very great service.

The principle of homeopathy he developed involves using the smallest effective dose of any medicine, which certainly is a reasonable proposition. Those who practice homeopathy look at the "symptom picture," which is the big picture or an appraisal of the entire person's physical, mental, and social makeup. The treatment often consists of very small doses of various medicines, many of herbal origin, for each physical or mental symptom. Starting a century ago, even smaller doses were used, below those that could produce a measurable effect in experimental observations by doctors. It is believed that these tiny doses do not directly attack the disease but stimulate the body's own defense activities; whereas larger doses may indeed paralyze defenses. This idea is not without precedent, as a similar effect was long ago observed in the action of nicotine on muscle contraction. Another theory of homeopathy is that "like cures like." This stands in contrast to the Eastern concept of opposites—yin and yang. If someday in the future successful homeopathic treatment should conflict with the theory behind it, there is ample precedent in orthodox medicine. As far as the patient is concerned, what works is what counts, not why it works.

The theory and practice of homeopathy spread to this country; by the middle of the nineteenth century there were over twenty schools of homeopathy in the United States. Hahnemann's name persists not only in the names of many hospitals throughout the country, but also in the name of a medical school in Philadelphia (which in recent years has for the most part given up any formal instruction in homeopathic medicine, perhaps to conform to the standard curriculum of other U.S. medical schools).

Recently the most intense increased interest has cropped up in Great Britain, where there has been much controversy aired in the scientific journal *Nature* regarding the theoretical and actual actions and results of the prescribed substances, which are increasingly diluted beyond measurable quantities.

There has been a recent resurgence of interest in homeopathy in the United States. In 1990 2.5 million Americans used homeopathic remedies, according to Dr. Eisenberg's study. A 1990 *Time* magazine poll revealed that 7.5 million Americans had seen homeopathic physicians. There are fewer than 500 physicians nationwide who describe themselves primarily as homeopaths, listing themselves as such in the Yellow Pages. Sales of homeopathic remedies, of which there are more than 1,200, are going up at the rate of 25 percent a year, totaling some $165 million a year at present, according to Jay Borneman, spokesman for the American Homeopathic Pharmaceutical Association. As of 1995, only three states, Connecticut, Nevada, and Arizona, had separate licensing boards for homeopaths. This compares with eight states that license naturopathic physicians (who usually have had some sort of traditional medical training) with added study in homeopathy, herbal medicines, acupuncture, and nutrition. As to testing the competency of homeopathic physicians, there is no agreement at this time. According to writer Judy Foreman, there are three separate boards that certify homeopaths according to their training.

CHIROPRACTIC

A more controversial but popular therapy is called chiropractic. Chiropractic is derived from the Greek words for "hand" and "effective." The theory behind chiropractic is that the nervous system integrates all body functions, including immunity. According to this theory many, if not most, ailments are caused by maladjustments of the spine. Even a slight movement of the openings in the spinal column through which the spinal nerves emerge to course throughout the body is called a "subluxation," and this may produce bodily changes that are painful or harmful. ("Luxation" means "dislocation"; "subluxation" implies a partial, perhaps undetectable, dislocation.) After the chiropractor has conducted a careful physical examination and perhaps X rays, the treatment consists of various kinds of massage or "adjustments." Practitioners claim success in treating lower back pain, slipped discs, and arthritis, but also in treating such apparently unrelated ailments as hay fever and high blood pressure. Chiropractors may or may not be licensed to prescribe drugs; the authorization to do so varies according to the legal requirements of individual states.

The concept of chiropractic originated in this country with David Palmer in 1895. Three years later he started his College of Chiropractic. At present there are over 30,000 practicing chiropractors, and they train in sixteen colleges, which may now have as many as 10,000 students taking the four-year course after high school, or sometimes two years of college. All states, except Mississippi and Louisiana, license chiropractors, and in all states they must pass a basic science examination. The training and standards for chiropractic are variable. Anybody contemplating use of chiropractic should ask the state organization for information and the state licensing board for details on requirements for training and licensing.

The American Medical Association for many years vigorously opposed chiropractic and cast doubt on its theoretical background, not only for reasons of competition, but also because chiropractic seems to call orthodox medical dogma into question. There have been, the AMA and others have pointed out, documented incidences of serious injury produced by chiropractic manipulation, but on the whole most patients seem to be satisfied. Grateful patients include some legislators who are not admirers of the established medical system. There are constant efforts to broaden the scope of practices legally permitted to be carried out by chiropractors.

As we have said, back pain and neck pain are among the com-

monest ailments treated by chiropractors; even with the most dili-
gent modern technologies the cause of such conditions is not always clear. Certainly treatment aimed at the supposed cause is not
always effective. Critics of chiropractic caution patients to be wary
of practitioners who recommend spinal treatments for conditions
that have nothing to do with spinal disease or injury, and they
warn that spinal manipulation can be dangerous for people with
spinal cord or brain injury. However, more and more practitioners
of chiropractic seem to be merging into the mainstream of health
care in this country. A large number of hospitals throughout the
United States now have freestanding chiropractic departments.

OTHER SYSTEMS

There are many other less well known and less widely practiced
systems of treatment. One is *reflexology*, a system based on the idea
that pressure applied to the feet and sometimes the hands promotes
a beneficial response throughout the entire body. There are also
healing systems built upon color therapy, dance therapy, art therapy, and music therapy. Whether or not the believed effectiveness
of these methods led to the formation of a theory or whether these
methods proceeded from application of a theory is hard to say.

Physical Treatment Systems

Many alternative therapies are based on physical intervention,
such as the laying on of hands.

At present the exercise fad in this country represents a happy
fusion of the beliefs of medical researchers, particularly with regard
to preventing cardiovascular disease, and the popular, almost fa-
natical, devotion to youth and "fitness." Books, videos, television
classes, and magazine advertisements have combined to produce a
lucrative industry. Many people find that exercise gives them a

sense of vigor and of self-worth. It may also help alleviate anxiety and depression. Various types of exercises promoted in health clubs and on television and in home videos have assumed large proportions as regulators of health and even as remedies for various ailments. In most cases the recommended exercises are aerobic exercises. "Aerobic" implies benefit from achieving elevation of the respiratory and pulse rates for a certain period of time, usually between twenty and thirty minutes. The implication is that the heart, lungs, and muscles will become stronger as a result of regular vigorous exercise. The evidence for the beneficial effects of regular moderate exercise is utterly convincing, but extreme exercise and the development of huge muscles has no proven long-term benefit.

Some techniques may involve what appears to be the opposite of vigorous exertion. For instance, yoga and tai chi involve postures, breathing techniques, and dancelike movements. At their best, both exercise and relaxation can be achieved at little or no expense. Recreational walking and running are the modern-day equivalents of the hard, manual labor that most people throughout the world have had to do throughout the ages. The late, great cardiologist Dr. Paul Dudley White was fond of pointing out that when he was a young doctor, coronary heart disease was virtually unheard of in the hospitals, particularly among men, most of whom did manual labor for twelve hours a day, six days a week. The public, in a strange twist of fate, now often pays money to achieve an end for which their forefathers received payment.

MASSAGE

Massage as a pleasurable form of relaxation and of relief from various kinds of neuromuscular complaints has ancient origins. Massage therapies of various sorts are practiced by people with widely varied levels of training and expertise, and in almost all societies in all countries. A partial list of types of massage therapy include:

acupressure, amna, body-mind centering, body-oriented psychotherapy, Chi Nei Sang, the Feldenkrais method, Jin Shin Do, the
Driya approach, massage therapy, neuromuscular therapy, Nuat thia,
Okazaki, Oriental bodywork therapies, polarity therapy, Reiki, rolf-
ing, shiatsu, the Trager approach, and Tuina. Within reasonable
limits of gentleness, massage, regardless of the theory employed or
the beliefs of the therapist, is almost always beneficial.

At present there are so many varieties of massage therapy available that most consumers are confused. Licensing of massage centers
by local boards of health or other health authorities is not universal, and such regulatory agencies are not able to obtain or provide
detailed, objective descriptions. A common practice for new patients
is to require that the therapist show evidence of four hundred to
five hundred hours of practice, supervised by a teacher certified by
one of the appropriate professional organizations, notably the American Massage Therapy Association. The workplace of the therapist
is usually subject to periodic inspection, but there is no way to control practice for home visits. For that reason massage therapists, like
hairdressers, are in many communities not permitted to work in
"clients'" homes.

Massage therapies of various sorts are practiced by people with
widely varied levels of training and expertise in the healing arts.
For instance, most acupuncturists combine the use of acupuncture
techniques with massage therapies.

HYDROTHERAPY

Another physical approach to treatment outside of the traditional
medical system is hydrotherapy, the use of hot or cold baths, sprays,
and immersion. Many of these treatments were part of mainstream
medicine in the nineteenth century. Treatment by immersion in or
even by drinking mineral or mud waters arising from deep in the
earth is not as popular in America as in Europe, but it has its strong

advocates. The craze for hot tubs has perhaps reached its peak, but more Americans than ever are installing jacuzzi baths in their homes with results that are gratifying to them in terms of well-being although it would be difficult to prove cost-effectiveness in terms of illness prevention.

There are, of course, other less widely used and less well known schools of health care and treatment. A sense of history is helpful in adopting the view that some of these therapies will almost certainly become incorporated into the mainstream health-care system in the future, but most of the others will disappear from sight perhaps only to reappear later, perhaps in a different guise. The future is never predictable. In this time of great turmoil in the health-care scene, most doctors of medicine seem to have come to an understanding and agreement that there are other ways of thinking and, indeed, other ways of treating people successfully. Most have dropped their vehement opposition. Osteopathy is a case in point.

In the nineteenth century there was competition between types of medicine taught in medical schools awarding M.D. degrees. As a result of this struggle, osteopathy was violently opposed by the American Medical Association for almost a hundred years, and has become progressively more regulated, organized, and involves more extensive training. Osteopaths practice essentially the same type of care as do M.D.'s but usually with more emphasis on physical-therapy types of treatment, such as the use of craniosacral treatments. Today the Doctor of Osteopathy (D.O.) in most communities and in many hospitals is on a par with the traditional M.D.

Likewise many of the options for alternative treatment of a wide variety of ailments will certainly continue to expand, probably to everyone's benefit. Useless and harmful practices will be more and more identified and eliminated. Training programs will be scrutinized and improved, and practitioners will be held to more stringent standards. It is human to turn away, perhaps in anger, from a doctor or health-care system that has failed to provide relief or to produce a cure, but it is not wise to plunge into new waters without gathering as much information as possible. The studies of alternative types of healing in medical schools and in the NIH will surely prove helpful.

9

Some Special Problems

*The recognition of the existence of a problem
is the first step in its solution.*

MARTIN H. FISCHER

No one can anticipate all of the health problems that may arise in life. In fact, trying to imagine every possible mishap is not natural to most of us and not good for anyone's mental health. There are some medical conditions, however, that commonly cause stress and confusion. If you have a predisposition for a certain ailment, or you worry about the effects of aging, it helps to think about your concerns in advance, preferably discussing with your doctor those symptoms that are bothering you at present or that you anticipate facing in the future.

Aging and the Care of Aging Relatives

HEALTH CONCERNS FOR THE ELDERLY

The number of people over sixty-five years of age will triple by the year 2024. Older people average eight visits per year to their physicians. People are living longer, and as they age some of their health problems and symptoms may be quite different from what they have been used to experiencing. For example, in addition to the obvious physiological changes, the elderly have different reactions to drugs than do younger patients. It is sometimes hard to tell the difference between the normal effects of aging and the effects of illness. The elderly may also develop fewer symptoms than younger people of some nonetheless serious underlying conditions. Appendicitis in the aged may be virtually free of pain until well advanced. I first learned this as an intern, when a patient being treated for arthritis on the hospital ward complained one day of only moderate abdominal pain; by that time the appendix had already ruptured.

We tend to think of old people in stereotyped ways, but in fact they are heterogeneous. Everyone knows of people who are active in every way into their nineties, and also people who in their early sixties are feeble in mind and body. Normal aging is gradual and never abrupt. Abrupt onset of symptoms almost always means there is a disease process present, but there is an almost universal tendency to overlook changes that may be significant. Geriatrics—the study and care of the aged—is one justifiably expanding medical specialty. Geriatricians have contributed enormously to our knowledge of the normal changes involved in aging and of the differences in response elderly people have to various illnesses and drugs.

Cultural differences may be as important as generational differences in producing friction when old people are living with their families. In matriarchal societies, where the mother has always ruled supreme at home, an autocratic grandmother can be a universal irritant as she continues to carry out her role unconsciously. The grandmother or grandfather who has been accustomed to acting as head of the family finds it hard to give up autonomy and resents being pushed into a passive, accepting role.

Certain physiological changes occur as one ages. These have been categorized as progressive loss of homeostatic reserve, which means that the ability of the body to keep things in balance is compromised. The body has a higher proportion of fat, and the lungs are stiffer, moving less air. Blood pressure tends to increase, although usually not to a dangerous degree. Muscles are weaker, bones are lighter and more easily fractured, and the brain shrinks in volume. Vision and hearing are diminished; 50 percent of people have significant loss of hearing by the age of seventy-nine. The thyroid very often begins to put out less of its hormone, and hypothyroidism among the aged is often underdiagnosed. Kidney function also tends to deteriorate. The adjustments of the heart and blood vessels to changes in position and pressure are diminished so that many old people may feel dizzy on suddenly sitting or standing, creating the possibility of dangerous falls. Immunity to most infectious diseases is generally diminished. Bacterial pneumonia is a much more dangerous disease among the elderly. For women who are not on hormone replacement, atrophy of the vaginal tissues may produce considerable discomfort, and they may become more prone to coronary heart disease than women receiving hormones. The level of the male hormone testosterone may decline in men as young as fifty, but in others it may remain relatively normal into the eighties. Loss of sexual desire, and loss of the ability to achieve an erection or orgasm, can cause older men to feel frustration and a sense of being less of a man, "over-the-hill." When one of a happily married couple loses the desire or capacity for sexual activity, depression and discord can occur. The sexual desires of old men often arouse disgust or scorn, further humiliating the man, who feels misunderstood. One older patient of mine, a thrice-married and lively woman, told me that she would be cheerfully ready to die when her days of vigorous sexual activity came to an end.

Noncancerous enlargement of the prostate and shrinking of the bladder capacity may produce problems with frequent urination and incontinence among men. Insomnia is a well-known feature of old age. Typically the sleep is less deep and is interrupted by frequent periods of wakefulness. These are all expected physiological changes. A popular bumper sticker proclaims OLD AGE IS NOT FOR SISSIES. Except for some wry humor, most people accept these losses with resignation and with courage.

There are some diseases and ailments, however, that are not normal or expected physiological responses. The most serious one is dementia, or loss of mental capacity. Alzheimer's disease is probably the leading cause, although the diagnosis can only be proved with certainty at present by a biopsy of brain tissue. Alzheimer's disease appears to be increasing in frequency, and, indeed, after the age of eighty it is extremely common. The fear of the possibility of memory loss is almost universal as people get older. The loss of memory for names is a normal occurrence with aging, but many older folks worry that it means they are developing Alzheimer's.

Depression is also common among the elderly, but it is not inevitable, and it does respond in most cases to suitable treatment. Incontinence of urine in either sex can frequently be helped or even cured by appropriate diagnosis and treatment. Immobility due to stiffness of the muscles and joints produces its own troubles: bedsores, loss of responsiveness resulting in falls, and loss of muscle strength. Most drugs are more slowly metabolized (physiologically changed within the body) or excreted more slowly by the elderly, so the usual adult dosages need to be decreased.

Older people, particularly those living alone and on a limited budget, are remarkably prone to malnutrition, which again is a highly correctable condition if identified. People who are neglected and isolated, either because there are no caring family members around or because they are in large institutions, deteriorate mentally and physically. Everyone needs stimulation and human interchange.

Lastly, there is something that happens to old people that is most unpleasant to consider, and that is abuse. Some people are abused in nursing homes or in large state institutions, but equally they may be abused at home by their own contemporaries, such as spouses, or by younger members of the family who resent the burden an elderly relative imposes. The abuse may take the form of verbal insults and put-downs, but all too often old people are beaten. Experienced workers in emergency rooms have come to recognize that injuries to old people are sometimes not caused by accident but by willful behavior, despite the statements by patients or caretakers on admission.

CARING FOR THE ELDERLY

To take care of old people who are experiencing some of these common impairments requires patience, a virtue that seems to be beyond the capacity of some people. Fortunately there are many who really enjoy working with and taking care of old people, for which all too often they receive no thanks. It has been said that one measure of the level of civilization of a society is the way in which it cares for old people. Knowing what to expect as a matter of course in aging can make the process easier for each of us.

Nursing-care facilities have expanded along with the aging population. There were 1.2 million nursing-home beds in 1971, and as of 1994 there were 1.9 million beds. The number of persons served by Medicare has risen from 16.27 million in 1980 to 25.1 million in 1991. More old people are living alone or with their spouses, or in some cases with their children, than are living in nursing care facilities. Living in the extended family was the usual pattern for old people until the 1940s. Today there are more households in which both spouses work, so no one is at home to care for a disabled older person. Other options for caring for elderly relatives need to be pursued. Because there is no tax-supported provision for long-term health-care insurance, there are not many health insurance options available. There are a few life-insurance companies, such as AMEX, Bankers Life & Casualty, Continental Casualty, or The Travelers, that do offer this rather expensive, but in many cases, extremely useful coverage. At present, people for the most part must pay for home health care and nursing-home care out of savings, earnings, or pensions.

Whether old people live alone, at home with family, or in nursing-care facilities, caregivers can be enlisted to ensure that they remain safe and healthy and happy. The nursing or health-care facility intake interview is important particularly when the interviewer cares and shows that he or she cares and is respectful to the patient. One widely used way of tracking the progress of elderly people is to keep track of the Activities of Daily Living (ADL). Changes in the daily living pattern indicate that something is wrong—sometimes major, sometimes minor. Home visits by a physician, nurse practitioner, or staff worker will often give valuable insights into the changes of the ADL that could not necessarily be obtained in an office visit or telephone call. Taking care of old people is often wearing, monotonous, and thankless work, so it is important to give respite to the caregivers. Health-care providers in many communities can put you in touch with a respite program, sponsored by hospice organizations, in which the old person is taken care of for a week or two, or maybe an evening or a weekend, while the caregiver gets a chance to have a break.

Talking to the very old can be a rewarding experience if a person can and will give the time. Unless the patient is quite deaf, it is better not to yield to the common tendency to shout. Caregivers should show respect, perhaps by not being too familiar in the use of a first name, and by waiting for a reply instead of impatiently repeating a question. I have often found with elderly patients that they at first appear not to have heard the question, or not to understand it. However, a brief, polite pause more often than not elicits a carefully thought out and rational response; it may be that it merely takes the older person a longer time to process a question and formulate a reply.

Although the great majority of people lose some of their hearing as they age, they often either do not realize that they are missing what is said or else choose to deny their hearing loss. The reason for this behavior was explained to me once by a wise, experienced audiologist who was testing my hearing, when I asked why people resist the idea of wearing a hearing aid. She pointed out that whereas eyeglasses may be needed even by the very young, that almost universally deafness is considered a sign of aging. With our American trait of hoping for eternal youthfulness, it is easier to accuse one's friends and family of mumbling than to acknowledge hearing loss. Wearing a properly adjusted and comfortable hearing aid has made life better for millions of people, but there remain many who for various reasons hate using them.

An elderly relative of mine many years ago seemed one day to be saying "what" particularly often. I said, "Where is your hearing aid?" "In the desk drawer," she replied. "Why?" I asked. "Because," she said tartly, "it keeps me from interrupting." This somewhat quirky reply showed in a few words the fierce desire for independence, the resentment of the inevitable losses of aging, and the insight and self-deprecating humor of so many old people. Understandably they resent being treated as dull witted or incompetent, as so often happens. Look at the messages in almost all birthday cards on display: when they depict aging they usually emphasize weakness, forgetfulness, wrinkles, flabbiness, and impotence. What does that tell us about our innermost feelings?

In the present political and economic climate it is not likely that there will be any increase in tax-supported housing and support for care of the elderly. The American Association of Retired Persons (AARP) lobbies hard in Washington to prevent cutbacks in the entitlements already in place, but the forces trying to reduce spending on the elderly are in power at this time. We should, therefore, all prepare not only to assist in the care of elderly relatives, but to plan for our own futures. In selecting a physician or a health plan, look for statements explaining their attitude toward old people, evidence of particular training in geriatrics, and especially their reputation for caring and consideration among older community members.

Women's Health Issues

In the great period of scientific advances in American medicine from 1890 to 1980, women's health was given little attention when it came to research and allocation of resources, and the great textbooks of medicine did not give women's health equal consideration. Actually for fifty years up to the year 1900 there was a higher proportion of women doctors in America than in subsequent times. During the period from 1900 to 1960 the number of women in medicine increased only slightly. In their struggle for recognition, academic advancement, and equality there was little progress. In the past four decades, women have become increasingly assertive in stating their needs and asking for greater resources. The impulse came largely from the women's movement rather than from within the medical profession. The first edition of the paperback *Our Bodies, Our Selves*, compiled by members of the Boston Women's Health Collective, was a landmark, and the book has since gone through many editions. Now every sizable bookstore has many titles relating to women's health. There is still a lot of progress to be made in diagnosis, research, and treatment. Unfortunately, the demands for equal recognition and care still meet with resistance, conscious or unconscious, in the male medical culture. The ever-increasing number of women graduating from medical school brings the promise of a more equitable distribution of resources and effort.

The differences between men and women go far deeper than sexual function, strength, and stature. Women may be prone to certain diseases and conditions because of physiology. To begin with, heart disease due to hardening of the coronary arteries was for years treated as if it were an exclusively male ailment. Research and treatment were accordingly slanted, and the diagnosis of heart disease due to narrowing of the coronary arteries has been, and still is, overlooked in women, whereas in fact it is the leading cause of death among older women, ranking above cancer.

Cancer of the breast now afflicts (according to various statistics) from one-in-nine to one-in-twelve women in this country, and the incidence may well be increasing. The overall rate of survival, while better than fifty years ago, is still not markedly different. There are two forms of cancer of the uterus, cancer of the cervix, or neck of the uterus, and cancer of the endometrium, or lining. The former undoubtedly has a viral component and may be related to the number of sexual partners a woman has had. Cancer of the cervix may be diagnosed by a Pap smear at an early stage, but the disease even then may progress rapidly, and is far less curable than endometrial cancer. It still has a high mortality rate. Cancer of the endometrium may well be accentuated by the widespread use of estrogens. Early detection and prompt treatment has made the prognosis (outlook) much better. In the case of both of these cancers, free access to careful gynecological examinations and use of the Pap smear to detect the presence of cancerous cells have been sadly underutilized, although the figures are improving. In this respect managed-care organizations have come to realize that preventive care can increase their profits over time by preventing costly later illness. Many of the managed-care plans have led the way in preventive approaches. For example, I have seen detailed printouts from one HMO listing patients who, according to their payment records, have not had the appropriate cholesterol, breast cancer, or Pap smear screening within the period suggested by the plan's guidelines.

Cancer of the lung, formerly primarily a male disease, is also increasing among women. This trend is undoubtedly related to the fact that as cigarette smoking has decreased among males, it has increased among younger women.

Violence is a particular health burden for many women. Because women fear to report it and because prosecutors and courts have been slow to recognize it, and reluctant to take action, domestic violence continues virtually unchecked. One woman in three is subject to physical violence at some time in her life, more often than not at the hands of a spouse, lover, or family member. The causes of this violence are not clear at this time, although a disproportionate number of violent acts take place when either the assailant or the victim is under the influence of alcohol. Women traditionally fear reprisal if they "tell," and, indeed, the published reports of batterers who continue to batter despite restraining orders, not to mention those who eventually kill their wives or girlfriends, seems to be increasing, certainly not decreasing.

Rape is another form of violence, and it is practiced primarily by men on women victims. The initial effects of rape may come from battering, bruising, suffocating, or stabbing. Sad to say, this is not the end of the damage suffered by the rape victim: depression, poor self-image, unwanted pregnancy, anxiety and guilt, as well as anger and fear persist for years, and call for support by therapists or organized support groups.

When primary-care doctors or nurses inquire about the possibility of abuse—mental, verbal, physical, or sexual—a woman has nothing to gain by concealing information. If a woman has been socialized to be passive, accepting, and not outspoken, as have most older women and members of some cultures, telling what has happened and asking for help may be difficult, but it is essential. Sensitivity training on these painful issues is available now to all medical personnel as well as police, but societal attitudes are somewhat slower to change.

Hypertension (high blood pressure) has no particular gender preponderance among women per se, but among African-American women it is very common, more common than among white women or black men. The reasons for this disparity are not known, but it may relate to variations between races in the regulation of salt by the kidney at a very early age.

Osteoporosis (loss of calcium from the bones) may occur in some women prior to menopause, but is much more common afterward. It is primarily a female disease often with a strong hereditary component. Attempts to treat it by hormones over the last fifty years have been disappointing. A woman with a strong family history of broken bones, particularly among her female relatives, probably should have bone-density studies and consultation with an expert in the field, as to the advisability of using estrogens and calcium. New medical treatments being introduced are promising, but, at present, the best one can be sure of is to prevent further bone loss, rather than to restore bone density to its normal level. Newly introduced pharmaceuticals seem in many cases to increase bone density. You should discuss this with your doctor.

As recorded in visits to medical facilities, depression is more common among women than men, as are anxiety disorders and the eating disorders including bulimia and anorexia nervosa. How many of these differences are gender related and how much of the depression and eating disorders relate to the expectations society places on women and to their treatment in a male-dominated society remains to be sorted out.

Women make more visits to doctors than men do, and they have more bedridden disabilities at home or in hospitals; nevertheless they consistently live longer than men, in every country. Taking these differences into account, a woman needs to be aware of some of the obstacles to care. The first is that there is too little information among health-care workers as well as the general public about the differences between male and female health risks. The second is that the availability of contraceptive advice, contraceptive options, and abortion has become increasingly politicized. Neither a health-care plan, managed or otherwise, nor a clinic should ever consider that it has a mandate to be a moral arbiter. We can only hope that laws will not be passed forbidding doctors in managed-care plans to discuss reproductive and other matters with their patients. When picking a health plan or a doctor, a woman needs to find out about the availability of the services she might require and the doctor's or plan's attitude toward reproductive health issues.

Early pregnancy deserves special consideration. The public should be educated that women who are pregnant need to consult a doctor at the earliest possible stage, as supervision and testing at the early stages of pregnancy make a large difference in the outcome. Women who are underage, uninsured, and unmarried frequently receive medical attention only when they go into labor, often with disastrous results. Surely one of the most important objectives of any health-care system, reformed or otherwise, should be the widespread availability of good prenatal care.

A woman needs to know as early as possible in her pregnancy what obstetrical services are available under her health plan. Doctors increasingly belong to group practice teams; a woman may not necessarily see the same obstetrician twice during a pregnancy, and she cannot be sure who is actually going to be present at the delivery. Many obstetrical practices in most states employ nurse-midwives, and in some states midwives are even permitted to practice as independent individuals. Many women prefer to have midwives as their primary obstetricians. Nurse-midwives are usually required to have an affiliation with an experienced obstetrician for consultation in difficult cases. It is also best for a woman to know whether she will be pushed out of the hospital within twenty-four hours of delivery.

Another obstacle that women, and men as well, must sometimes overcome is bureaucratic resistance to changing doctors or seeking a specialist within a health-care plan. The choice of a doctor is a highly personal matter; the patients' preferences sometimes do not receive the consideration they deserve. Women clearly need the maximum of information before choosing a health-care plan or physician, but according to the nature of one's particular managed-care plan there may be little or no choice. When choice is available, however, the gender of a woman's primary-care physician may be extremely important, but even more important is whether or not the physician is a sympathetic listener. As mentioned before, there are no hard and fast rules telling how to proceed with this choice. Health-care plans usually have a list of primary-care providers; the patient has to do considerable calling around, looking up qualifications and references, and some leg work to get the descriptive and personal reports of the available physicians. These reports are understandably subjective; the first choice of physician may not turn out to be the best one, so knowing the rules for changing physicians within the health plan also becomes important.

Managed-care plans sometimes penalize women by making referrals to specialists in fertility, osteoporosis, and issues of hormone-replacement therapy difficult since these services add to the costs of the plan. The woman is left with trying to solve her problems with a primary-care doctor who does not have expertise in these fields. Also, as noted, women appear to have a higher incidence than men of some depression and anxiety states, although not of major psychoses. For that reason women may have more difficulty than men in receiving referrals for psychotherapy.

A woman may have difficulty arriving at certain decisions crucial to her health because of conflicting advice from various authorities. Some of these issues, discussed below, are the advisability of hormone-replacement therapy, early-detection tests for breast cancer, and treatment courses for breast cancer. Organizations such as the American College of Obstetricians and Gynecologists (ACOG), the American Cancer Society (ACS), and the American College of Physicians (ACP) have from time to time issued recommendations in the form of position papers; many women's organizations have also taken positions on some of these difficult decisions. It seems that almost every issue of the major women's magazines has an article on decisions in women's health. Most of these are reliable and informative, but in the long run each woman still has to make the decision herself. It is in this situation that a good relationship with a caring and experienced family physician is most useful.

Hormone-Replacement Therapy (HRT)

The pros and cons of using estrogens with or without progestin at and after menopause have been and will undoubtedly remain for a long time controversial and emotional. One way to lessen the anger or anxiety surrounding this decision to some extent is by taking the advice of a female expert in this field, which has until recently been long dominated by men. There are many excellent works now available for women, so women should take the opportunity to become familiar with the arguments for and against each position. In HRT the use of estrogens with or without progestins seems to keep the vaginal and vulvar tissues from senile atrophy, may prevent bone loss (osteoporosis), and probably is protective against coronary heart disease. Such arguments must be balanced against an increased risk of endometrial cancer and possibly, but not proven, an increased risk of breast cancer with HRT.

Early Detection of Breast Cancer

Early detection of breast cancer is facilitated by frequent (annual or semiannual) mammograms combined with a program of regular self-examination and examination by a physician. The question is at what age are routine mammograms recommended. The statistics on the value of routine mammograms below a certain age, variously placed between twenty and thirty-five, are confusing. The results of early detection are real but not impressively encouraging. Managed-care plans try to set standards and guidelines for these examinations for monetary reasons, but in any case predictability is uncertain. Each woman needs to consider her own risk factors: breast cancer in the case of her mother or maternal grandmother, obesity, smoking, a high-fat diet, and possibly the use of estrogens are risk factors. In the end personal preferences, the opinion of peers, and published statements, can all contribute to making the final decision. Some family doctors will make firm recommendations, but others will try only to present the facts as far as they can be determined, leaving the decision to the patient. The fear of accusations of malpractice casts a shadow over the doctor who might offer well-meaning advice. The financial pressures driven by fear of not being covered for some procedures of uncertain merit should not, but in real life actually do, affect a woman's decision.

Treatment of Breast Cancer

Conservative, radical, or unconventional treatment are choices breast-cancer patients face. This is truly a field for experts. Hundreds, even thousands of research reports compete for attention and acceptance. Surgery, radiation, and chemotherapy are the mainstays of treatment, but how much and what type of each is always a matter of debate. After all the options are presented to the patient, she must add to the mix her own feelings about mutilation, pain, and the prolongation of suffering. Support from caregivers and family is crucial at this time. Cancer patients in many centers are helped by joining groups for mutual support and discussion. The distressing and often bleak outlook sends many people to seek alternative therapies, including various "natural" healing pathways. The difficulty is that at present there seems to be no reliable objective assessment of the results of any of these treatments. Desperate people can hardly be faulted for exploring all those alternatives. To quote Samuel Johnson, taking such measures may represent "the triumph of hope over experience."

Routine Gynecological Exams

The ideal interval between routine gynecological checkups of a symptom-free woman is also unsettled. The recommendations of the American College of Obstetrics and Gynecology call for shorter intervals and a younger age at first visit than do the American Cancer Society, the American College of Physicians, and most health plans.

In larger group practices and health plans, routine gynecologic examinations are now often carried out by nurses. The results to date show a high rate of reliability and patient satisfaction. Statistically speaking, the doctor may not be essential, since a questionnaire as well as laboratory tests and examinations by nurses or technicians, impersonal as they may be, can identify many but not all risks. Some women are thus reassured, but others, perhaps most women, want the input of a doctor. It seems to me that almost all gynecological problems identified by a nurse practitioner or primary-care medical doctor should be dealt with by a board-certified gynecologist. But some conditions, such as yeast infections, may be well handled by a nurse or primary-care doctor. Most managed-care plans in group practices have guidelines specifying suggested management of common gynecological problems. It may well be that in the future, plans will not pay for highly specialized routine gynecological exams. Your health plan probably has guidelines that should be flexible enough to account for variations in risk factors.

Behavioral, Emotional, and Other Mental-Health Disturbances

Picking a doctor and a health plan is, as we know, complicated and difficult. When one is faced with the need to seek help for an emotional, interpersonal, substance-abuse, or mental-health problem, the choice is even more difficult. It may prove helpful to look back and see how we arrived at the present situation.

For the most part, until the late nineteenth century, unusual antisocial behavior was thought to be caused by a defect of character, sometimes the work of the devil, and sometimes due to sheer cussedness. As medicine began to take more rational approaches in the nineteenth and early twentieth centuries, psychiatry came into being as a recognized and accepted medical specialty and began attempts at classifying and treating mental-health problems. At the same time, spiritual healing, promoted by organized religion and irregular cults, flourished alongside of "rational" medicine. Psychiatrists were few in number and not well accepted by the general public or by the general medical profession until the era of World War II. In fact, until that time they were called "alienists," a term that reflected the public's fears and misconceptions. Freudian concepts thereafter permeated not only medical discussions but all aspects of life. Abnormal behavior of various sorts became medicalized. The poet Ezra Pound was committed to a federal mental hospital, not jailed as a traitor, for his radio broadcasts from occupied Italy during World War II. During the cold war, extreme attitudes and behavior offensive to the authorities were often treated as psychological aberrations, particularly in countries behind the Iron Curtain. In this country the trials of Whittaker Chambers and Alger Hiss, for example, became a platform for various widely publicized psychiatric pronouncements.

The high cost of prolonged psychotherapy was not, and still is not, covered by most forms of health insurance. People who were frankly psychotic were, and still are, for the most part taken care of in tax-supported mental hospitals. In the 1960s there was a change in the public attitude toward institutionalization, and the buzz-word in mental health was "deinstitutionalization." That meant that people would no longer be kept in large mental hospitals for long periods of time, but were discharged into the community supposedly in the care of their families and a network of ambulatory providers. The first part, that is, emptying out the hospitals, was carried out with dispatch, saving vast amounts of money. One of the advances in treatment that made this possible was the widespread introduction of antipsychotic drugs, of which Haldol is perhaps the best example. Unfortunately, the community and family support that the idealistic but unrealistic planners of the 1960s proposed never came into being, and as a result we have a large population of people sorely in need of mental-health counseling and even hospitalization who are living on the streets or are, sadly, in prisons.

In 1994 5.6 percent of the adult population, some 10.7 million persons, were treated for mental and/or addictive disorders in specialty clinics and hospitals, and another 6.4 percent, or 11.5 million persons, were treated in the general medical sector, but there are no reliable figures on the millions of people who go to other mental-health therapists. According to the U.S. Department of Health and Human Services, in 1994 schizophrenia accounted for the largest number of doctor and clinic mental-health visits. The next most common category was the affective disorders, notably bipolar or manic-depressive disorder. Eighty-five percent of mental-health contacts were in an ambulatory setting, and only 5 percent of patients were treated solely in mental hospitals. The remainder were treated with a combination of both inpatient and outpatient care. The spectrum of mental-health care ranges from total hospitalization to residential treatment care, thence to residential supportive or part-time care, thence to outpatient or ambulatory care.

As to inpatient treatment facilities, in 1980 there were 278 state mental hospitals in this country, but thirteen years later this number had fallen to 256, and forty-two states reporting to the government in 1993 announced plans to downsize their mental hospitals further. The total number of psychiatric beds available to the public in 1970 was 524,878; this figure fell in the next twenty years to 272,293. There are more private psychiatric or mental-health hospitals than state, tax-supported hospitals, although the private institutions tend to have fewer beds. In 1990 there were 466 private hospitals, and of their 42,000 beds only 62 percent were occupied.

Medicaid mental-health funds are administered by the individual states, so that eligibility, allowable length of stay, and so on, vary. For example, not all states reimburse psychiatric ambulatory-care services. Twenty-three states limit the number of reimbursable days for mental health.

The high cost of psychotherapy and disputes over the effectiveness of psychiatric treatment have encouraged legalization of many forms of therapy by practitioners who have received various levels of training and who adhere to various schools of belief; third-party payments are now restricted to short-term therapy and crisis management. Since third-party funding for the services of psychiatrists (M.D.'s) is rapidly shrinking under managed care, many psychiatrists have turned to full-time salaried work or other occupations entirely. Still other psychiatrists have concentrated on pharmacotherapy, prescribing tranquilizers, antidepressant drugs, and some of the newer antipsychotic drugs. Clinical psychologists, psychiatric social workers, and all other psychotherapists, who previously received third-party payments, are also experiencing now a smaller patient load, and they must charge their patients directly.

Where does this leave the person in need of mental-health therapy? For those who are able to pay out of pocket, there are many choices between therapists of some of the varieties discussed in chapter 3. For those who cannot pay, there are public clinics; they usually have long waiting lists, and therapists don't have sufficient time to spend with each patient. Therapy groups, either professionally led or self-perpetuating, have flourished under this system. Churches, YMCAs, YMHAs, women's groups, and some trade unions have, with varying degrees of success, organized mental-health support groups with professional leadership. Parents of children with school adjustment problems and severe behavior problems have turned either to private psychiatric help, poorly funded public clinics, or school guidance counselors, of whom there are relatively few who are well trained.

The primary-care physician in some managed-care organizations can assist the patient by selecting a psychotherapist and making the referral for a limited period of treatment based on a specific diagnosis. Increasingly, however, HMOs have a separate organization for referral and funding of mental-health consultations. The primary-care physician may have little or no input into the choice of therapists for his patient. The patient may be given a separate telephone number to call and then may have to negotiate with a triage (sorting) professional who decides which therapist the patient can see and how many visits will be paid for according to the presumed diagnosis. A good managed-care organization takes care to see that such therapists are well qualified professionally; of course, there is no guarantee that the patient and therapist will get along well or be a good fit.

Much of the responsibility for behavioral problems, therefore, comes back to the patient. There is a wide spectrum of behaviors and feelings that may be considered normal, and everyone has to consider for himself or herself whether certain thoughts and feelings are sufficiently out of the ordinary to require professional help. These judgments are often made by knowledgeable family members, by guidance counselors at school or work, or by clergy members. A primary-care physician who is interested, knowledgeable, and has the time to get to know the patient is probably the best resource for referral.

For those who are interested in reading in detail the professional classification of various forms of mental disorders, the *DSM IV* (Diagnostic and Statistical Manual), a multiauthored work developed over many years by the American Psychiatric Association, is not only helpful but surprisingly interesting reading. This work is also summarized in an easily readable descriptive shorter version that is available in most bookstores. Be warned, however, that it is sometimes hard to separate excessive self-analysis from necessary self-awareness. Socrates said that the unexamined life is not worth living, but the excessively examined life can be unproductive.

Adolescent Issues

As a family grows up, parents often are caught by surprise as their children become adolescents. Adolescents have a period of rapid growth, which occurs at about the age of twelve in girls and a year later for boys. During this time they develop the capacity for abstract thinking and start to form their goals in life, but most important they are struggling to identify themselves as independent individuals. Specialists in adolescent medicine are increasing in number and organization. Managed-care plans vary in their capacity to provide referral to such experts in cases that require treatment that is beyond the capacity of the plan's primary-care generalists.

Once, when a thirteen-year-old boy rebelled at having to go to a "baby doctor," his mother brought him to me as an internist, a "grown-ups' doctor." He was solemn and quietly polite during the history-taking and physical examination. At the conclusion I asked him to sit down for a summary. I told him how much he had gained in height and weight. I reassured him that all of his bodily systems were in excellent working order. This seemed to please him. Then I said: "And you are maturing nicely. Your voice is changing." He looked anxious for the first time and asked me, "Up or down?" This was his only revelation of the profound anxiety of the young adolescent in connection with sexual identity.

The health risks of adolescents in this country at this time are serious depression; substance abuse, including alcohol, drugs, and tobacco; injuries; the results of premature sexual activity; and the emergence of risk-taking behaviors, such as the ignoring of seat belts, refusing to wear helmets, and ignoring reasonable driving habits. At this time eating disorders often emerge so gradually, particularly among girls, that the parents are not aware until anorexia or bulimia have reached an advanced stage. One of the leading causes of death among adolescents is suicide. The risks are hard to identify, and there are occasionally clusters of suicides among adolescents that have the appearance of a contagious epidemic disease. Even the closest, most loving families are rudely surprised by the suicide attempt of an adolescent child.

Issues in the Care of Children

One of the more difficult decisions with which a parent is faced is whether to send a sick child to school and when to call the doctor or bring the child in for an appointment. As a general rule of thumb, sick children always belong at home. A sore throat or a cold, if mild, probably is not a bar to going to school, as it is impossible to keep away from school all those who have mild colds in the early stages, even though that is when colds are most contagious. Children with a fever of over 100 degrees should not be sent to school, nor should a child be sent to school who has an unusual skin rash, unless the doctor has indicated that this is safe. In your advance planning, be sure to arrange for a fallback plan for alternative care of your child or children if both parents are working.

Before calling the doctor on the telephone about a rash, make note of the location, color, and texture of the rash, when it began, and whether it was associated with fever. Similarly, be prepared to give the doctor accurate descriptions of other ailments such as colds, upset stomach, and diarrhea. The doctor or nurse practitioner should be able to give treatment advice about many common contagious diseases over the telephone. He or she usually knows what is epidemic in the area at that time. Vomiting and diarrhea are definite reasons not to permit the child to go to school.

Doctors, Sexual Preference, and Gender Issues

Discussions between doctor and patient are nowhere more important than in the area of issues of sexuality. Sex education in America is backward compared with that of most other developed countries. Embarrassment and prudishness often prevent parents from helping their children develop an informed and mature attitude toward sexuality. Not only parents but doctors should become comfortable in discussing these issues. It is never easy for a parent or a doctor to decide when it is the proper time to talk about sex with their children and patients. Most parents procrastinate until it is too late to be informative and supportive to their children. Those who most vehemently oppose sex education in school often state that providing such information encourages early experimentation and promiscuity. There is no credible proof of this claim. Sexuality is inborn and cannot be made to go away. Television, movies, magazines, and all advertising combine to thrust awareness of sex on all children at an early age.

Gays, lesbians, and bisexuals want and deserve physicians, nurses, and a medical system familiar with their problems and sympathetic, or at the very least, nonjudgmental of them and their health problems and risks. Younger physicians are perhaps more likely to meet these criteria since they are more likely to come from colleges and graduate schools where open acceptance and discussion of different life choices have been increasingly common. Even so, homophobia is still common at all levels of society and is sometimes expressed with open hostility. Hospitals operated by religious orders tend to have a less-accepting attitude. Because of widespread prejudice, many homosexuals seek medical care in clinics and offices that are known to be knowledgeable as well as sympathetic, although they may not be covered by health insurance. Every metropolitan-area telephone book lists some gay and lesbian groups that can give appropriate medical referrals. There are, in some places such as libraries and schools, legal constraints on discussing homosexuality or a more open sexual lifestyle; although to date physicians and nurses are not forbidden to give such advice, legislation curtailing the dissemination of information has been proposed.

A good pediatrician takes time to discuss with parents and children sexual issues, not for the purpose of moralizing, but for the purpose of educating them so patients can know themselves and protect themselves. The deep anxieties over sexual identity that worry many, if not most, growing children are natural and are only intensified when discussion is avoided. When a clear-cut homosexual preference emerges, the doctor, parents, and patient need to talk about the future, how to avoid health risks, and acceptance of sexuality. Established homosexuality probably has strong biological roots and cannot be "cured," so it shouldn't it be treated as a remediable illness. Ideally, managed-care practices should have a staff sympathetic to differences in lifestyles and orientations, but unfortunately this is not always the case.

In the matter of choosing a doctor, these are all subjects on which you may want to sound out your primary-care physician early in your acquaintance.

Fatal Diseases: Death and Dying

If we in America are reluctant to face and talk openly about sexuality, we are perhaps even more reluctant to face and openly discuss the possibility or inevitability of death. Doctors from the beginning of their education are confronted with death as a reality, but, surprisingly enough, many doctors avoid thinking about and discussing death, much to the detriment of their relationships with their patients. It has been suggested many times that one strong unconscious motivation for young people entering the field of medicine is to conquer death or at least to try to control it. But efforts are now being made in medical schools to foster in physicians a more realistic view of the end of life.

One of the matters you'll want to discuss with your doctor is your own attitude toward terminal illness. The living will is an instrument widely used but not legally binding in all states. This is a document signed at a time when the patient is well and of sound mind, and it in effect says that when all hope of recovery is gone, then painful, prolonged, and expensive treatment should be discontinued. Law offices and many hospitals and managed-care plans have copies of these forms available. The most important feature of a living will is that the people taking care of the patient know that it exists.

Patients with terminal illnesses are increasingly asked about their preferences. The immediate family likewise can express a preference in managing the last illness. The physician in charge discusses what may happen and the consensus of the family members and the patient. These decisions are then supposed to be written as an order in the hospital chart, but it does not always in real life work out the way it is intended. Sometimes the patient by words or actions indicates a change of heart and a desire to work with the powerful life force that exists within each of us, driving us to live on. Even more distressing are the times (which I and many other physicians have experienced) when family members are divided over the course of action. In a recent widely publicized lawsuit against a prominent Massachusetts hospital, one member of the family sued the physicians, the hospital, and a senior member of the hospital's ethics committee, because the patient had expressed a wish to be permitted to die, and all of the children, except this one had agreed with this course of action. The one dissenting member of the family brought suit with an accusation of wrongful death. The court decided against this plaintiff.

Another way in which the patient can express his or her wishes for the management of a last illness is through the so-called health-care proxy. As opposed to a living will, where the patient's prior wishes are involved and painful decisions need to be made by the immediate family, oftentimes by people who have a monetary interest in the outcome, with the health-care proxy, the decision-making role is ideally given to a disinterested party, but someone who has known the patient well, who sympathizes with the patient's outlook, and who accepts the serious obligation of carrying out these wishes at the appropriate time. Almost all American hospitals have written policies covering these matters. In the case of any serious illness the patient and the family should be aware that this policy exists and act accordingly.

There are some diseases for which the outcome is certain. The best known, at present, is AIDS, since there is no cure, although some lengthening of life is possible. Some kinds of cancer are incurable at the time they are discovered. The question always arises in such circumstances as to what the patient should be told, when, and by whom. Very often loving spouses or children plead that the patient not be told of a fatal diagnosis. At this time a family doctor with a good relationship with the patient and family is invaluable. A doctor has a legal as well as a moral obligation to give the diagnosis and prognosis to the family and, in the opinion of most who have dealt with the subject in depth, a moral obligation to tell the patient in the best way possible. After the tremendous initial shock of being told of the prognosis, most patients go through a period of grieving and very often of anger. In the long run the patient is better equipped to face the inevitable if he or she is told the whole truth. There are some points on which the doctor and the patient should be in agreement. This is not possible if the patient doesn't have all the facts. First, the diagnosis must be certain before any bad news is given. Second, the patient must be competent to understand the matter and to make conscious and reasonable decisions. Third, the patient has every right to refuse treatment, a right that was upheld by the U.S. Supreme Court in the Cruzan case. Advance directives such as the living will and the health-care proxy need to be consulted at this time.

Somehow caregivers must temper the bad news by giving hope. The hope need not be in the form of a promise that a cure might be possible, but hope can come from the assurance that there will be the least possible pain or suffering, that loved ones will be nearby, and that the doctor, indeed, cares and will be available. It is comforting to the patient to know that the doctor has a plan of action.

The patient, the family, and the primary-care doctor, having jointly decided how to manage the patient's last days or hours, face another important decision as to where the death should take place. Most people in the recent past traditionally have died in a hospital. Under managed care, terminal-care patients are generally either sent home or to some form of chronic-care or nursing-home facility. When by written agreement of all parties no treatment other than simple palliative measures are to be provided, the hospital is really not at all a good place for a person to die. The atmosphere is barren and unfamiliar. The same may be said of nursing-care facilities. Some enlightened managed-care plans provide financial support for home care in terminal illness, and this is perhaps the best solution, again provided that the diagnosis and prognosis are certain. Hospice care, where available, is an excellent solution. These agencies offer virtually every service offered by a hospital, other than surgery, and the cost and stresses of hospitalization for the patient are avoided. Such services are, as might be expected, expensive. Third-party payments are in many cases available. In some instances, Medicare or Medicaid will reimburse most of these costs for a limited time, but only after previous acute-care hospitalization. Commercial insurers in some cases offer such coverage; it is expensive and often incomplete, but nevertheless it is potentially a great help. At home, familiar faces and surrounding objects are at hand, the time of day or night is not regulated by institutional rules, and honest displays of emotion and affection and prayer seem more natural at home.

Hospice care is limited to patients who are not expected to live over six months. The doctor in charge of the case notifies the hospice organization, with the informed consent of the patient and the family, giving the diagnosis and the expectations (prognosis). The care is most often in the home of the patient. There are a limited number at this time of inpatient hospice facilities. The hospice has not only trained nurses available, but, more importantly, a number of trained and sympathetic volunteers. The bond between the patient and the helpers becomes very strong. Medication is limited to the relief of pain and suffering. Hospice nurses are permitted in most states to obtain and administer narcotics for the relief of pain.

Suicide brings out perhaps the strongest and most conflicting emotions of any form of death. The suicide of someone who is not intoxicated is the ultimate expression of a loss of hope. It almost always comes as a tremendous surprise as well as a shock to those who know the victim. Two immediate reactions inevitably occur. The first is a sense of guilt — "I wish I had known. Perhaps I could have helped"; the other reaction is an attempt to assign blame. Sometimes an obvious reason or cause appears that meets with general acceptance, but the sad fact is that the cause is very often not clear. What went on in the mind of the suicide victim before the event may never be known. Among the warning signs are an unpredictable and sudden change in behavior, including uncontrollable outbursts of anger, withdrawal from the usual activities with friends and family, insomnia at night with drowsiness or apathy by day, heavy consumption of alcohol, and preoccupation with firearms.

A primary-care doctor or nurse can sometimes identify risk factors for suicide and initiate intervention. The known risk factors have been widely discussed and documented, but they do not seem to be apparent in the case of many suicidal acts. Parents and teachers should nevertheless be vigilant for suicidal symptoms in teenagers. Feelings of lack of identity and self-worth are extremely common among adolescents. Events that intensify these feelings, such as general family hostility or severe punishment at school or in a court are powerful destroyers of fragile self-esteem. Although it is understandable that parents want their children to succeed, sometimes they put too much pressure on a child to be perfect and to live up to unrealistic expectations. Sometimes an intuitive primary caregiver can see this happening and discuss the problem with the family before it is too late. In a managed-care system the prevention of suicide through staff alertness can hardly be reduced to a set of treatment guidelines nor assigned a dollar value. The family should be able to get in touch with the primary caregiver when it is even remotely possible that an adolescent is contemplating suicide. In some cities there is a suicide hotline (often listed in the phone book under "Samaritans"), manned by volunteers who have been well trained in dealing with the situation.

10

Ready, Aim, Fire: Preparing, Choosing, and Making Your Moves

Suit the action to the word, the word to the action;
with this special observance, that you o'er step not
the modesty of nature.

WILLIAM SHAKESPEARE, *Hamlet*

Be Prepared to Face Some Tough Decisions

There comes a time when, after gathering as much information as possible, one must make decisions about future health care and put a plan into action. There are some health decisions that only you can make, and you must make them based on incomplete information. No one, no matter how diligently he or she studies and inquires, knows with certainty the "right" choice. A Chinese proverb says it well: "To be uncertain is uncomfortable, but to be certain is ridiculous." For example, after going to the primary-care doctor a woman past menopause must decide whether or not to use hormone-replacement therapy (HRT), usually estrogen with or without progestin. She must balance her own risks and concerns about the possibility of heart attacks or fractured bones, versus the possible side effects of the hormone—an increased risk of cancer of the uterus or even possibly of the breast. Very often a woman asks her primary-care doctor to make these decisions for her, but the physician, knowing the uncertainties involved and aware of the penalties for making wrong choices, is apt to tell the patient that the choice is hers to make; no one is very confident of having made the right choice.

To take another example, a conscientious mother, after reading many articles in newspapers and magazines, must decide how little saturated fat, such as butter, eggs, and cream to feed her children, to avoid the later development of coronary artery disease. Then she reads that an excessively low-fat diet may hinder the full development of the brain and hormone systems. Finally, a friend points out that the French who eat all the good forbidden foods have less heart attacks than Americans. Another friend compounds this by saying that the consumption of red wine by the French is what keeps them healthy, but the good mother is hesitant to push the regular use of red wine on her family. To confuse the decision-making process further, several cardiologists have written that red wine is conducive in some people to the aggravation of a dangerous disorder of the heart rhythm known as atrial fibrillation. The more medical reports are published and broadcast to the public, the more difficult it is to make decisions.

In another example, men in their sixties and seventies often lose their sexual potency and are found to have a low level of testosterone. Regular injections of this hormone may greatly improve sexual performance, satisfaction, even self-esteem. The downside is the increased possibility of cancer of the prostate gland. Once again, all of us must live with ambiguity. A decisive person will look at the facts available to him, choose one course, and not look back. Others are more thoughtful and more anxious and inevitably will rely on others to come to a decision. Sexual activity may be more important to some than others. Ideally there should be a family doctor, who knows not only the patient but his culture and his family, to help sway the decision. Such transactions need a lot of time; arranging this time with your doctor is a major stumbling block.

Yet another difficult decision that many people face is whether or not to continue every extreme measure including resuscitation to prolong the life of an unconscious or semiconscious patient suffering from a painful terminal illness. As previously mentioned, the living will and the health-care proxy made out in advance by the patient (everyone should be sure to make out one of these) is an excellent guide, but in some places the document is not legally binding. Euthanasia, the willful and intentional use of fatal treatment for a dying patient, is illegal in this country, although in limited form it is legal in the Netherlands. A family should never urge their doctor to commit such an act. Without any doubt, many physicians and other caregivers have in some manner made it easier for patients to die, usually by acts of omission rather than of commission. Physician-assisted suicide, which was recently legalized in Oregon but has been challenged in the courts, is another matter. An extensive discussion on physician-assisted suicide by a task force of the Society of Health and Human Values was issued in 1995. This comprehensive report does not advocate the practice, but it does list five topics and related questions physicians should ask themselves before establishing a policy on physician-assisted suicide. The commission also went on to study in depth the questions that a patient and a family must consider before even considering suicide.

Know Yourself

No one can be expected to make a reasonable approach to health care on insufficient information. Having gathered as much information as possible, it is even more important to weigh the importance of various factors. No two people have exactly the same values. Obviously, the most valuable but perhaps the most difficult task is knowing yourself. There will always be friends and family who will tell you what you should think or what you should do or what you are like, but in the end only you can know your innermost self.

There are a number of tasks you take on when you decide to take responsibility for your health care, including deciding what services you are apt to need, how you will react to potential health problems, and how everyday habits affect your health. Imagine various situations in which you may find yourself and how you would proceed in case of assault, fire, or natural disaster. Make an inventory of your health, of known risks to your health, of what you want and expect of your body. The strongest factor in anyone's health and longevity is heredity, about which at present we can do very little. It is crucially important to know the family history of coronary artery disease, high blood pressure, diabetes, cancer, particularly of the breast and uterus among women and of the prostate and digestive tract among men, and a strong family history of mental disorders, particularly the bipolar (manic-depressive) disorder. Alcoholism tends to run in families, members of which should periodically assess their own drinking habits and be particularly observant and supportive as their children enter adolescence. Fear is a force destructive to anyone's health, and it needs to be identified. Most people fear abandonment, assault, poverty, cancer, pain, and death itself. Facing up to one's fears and making appropriate plans for action is one of the greatest safeguards to health.

Assess your lifestyle and any associated health risks. Sort out proven allergies from things you simply don't like. Make conscious decisions about the risks and benefits to you of smoking, drinking, and drug use. Write these down and look at them several times subsequently, to see if you have been honest with yourself. Likewise, if you opt for promiscuous sexual behavior, this should be a conscious decision made while sober, weighing carefully the pros and cons in advance.

Everyone seems to talk today about stress as if this were a new and preventable epidemic. Life is, and always has been, full of stress. In a self-assessment one needs to identify not only the sources of stress, but especially one's own response to it. Many people thrive under stress, but for others stress may precipitate some skin diseases, allergies, depressions, temporomandibular joint syndrome, or painful menstruation. None of these conditions are purely the result of stress, and all of them can be faced by self-knowledge and with the help of your primary-care practitioner.

There are also some conditions that have current notoriety as threats to health and that need careful consideration. The chronic fatigue syndrome is still difficult to define and even more difficult to treat. Many people are worried that their blood sugar goes too high or too low, but this can be very easily ruled out by a simple blood test. Other people hear of systemic Monilia (yeast infection), but again the facts are hard to come by, and the diagnosis deserves a skeptical approach. PMS, the premenstrual syndrome, is a very real condition, but it is blamed for many situations for which it is not really responsible.

In assessing one's own health, it is hard to admit to some of the deepest fears, such as feelings of sexual inadequacy, abandonment, shyness, lack of self-confidence, and loneliness. Having faced the painful recognition of factors such as these, it may be even harder to find a sympathetic therapist in your health plan, or an affordable one outside the health plan.

Finally, no one's health exists in a vacuum. The effects of depression, alcoholism, and heavy drug use resonate throughout the entire family. The size of your family can be a source of friction and anxiety, ranging on the one end from the problems of infertility through consideration of contraception and abortion, and at the other end worry about a family too large to care for properly. Everyone who is concerned with health, from providers to sufferers, has a different idea of what to seek and what to avoid.

Everyone from time to time feels poorly. The great doctor William Osler once remarked that most of the work of this world is done by people who do not feel quite well. Americans are living longer, but it is unreasonable to expect immortality to or blame a person or thing for the death of an extremely ill or elderly person. Everyone who is older can count on moving more slowly, thinking more slowly, being stiff in the muscles and joints, probably a little bit deaf, and definitely more tired at the end of the day. This is something that everyone should expect and plan for so as not to be surprised by these symptoms. Excellent work is now being done by the one rapidly deservedly expanding specialty, geriatrics, to foster better health and activeness of older people. The reports of hormones or similar substances such as melatonin, which may delay some of the aging process, are exciting. The use of strong antioxidant vitamins, particularly vitamins C and E, is also promising, but much more research is needed to separate the facts from overblown advertising claims. A comfortable lifestyle, keeping active physically and mentally, eating and drinking moderately, nurturing friendships, and joining groups are all helpful strategies that do not require doctors and, in fact, help reduce the need to see the doctor.

Continuing the assessments that go into making up a health-care plan, consider one's spouse. A wife, bearing in mind her husband's heredity, needs to know if her husband is a macho denier of symptoms who will run past the danger signals of obesity, substance abuse, or any of the warning signs of serious illness. A husband needs to know his wife's biggest worries, and whether she is receiving the support she needs from health-care providers. Aging parents, whether they live with their adult children or not, are an increasingly common source of concern as well as a financial and emotional drain for many families. The children who are responsible for older parents need to know what resources are available in the community as well as what insurance provisions are available to them under Medicare and Medex. Ideally all members of the family from the youngest to the oldest should be involved in decision making. Young children who see their grandparents being treated in a sympathetic way will grow up to treat their own parents similarly.

Knowledge is power up to a point, but judgment is hard to learn. The fear of making a wrong decision should not interfere with the need to make some decision about your health. Robert Browning said, "The business of life is making terrible choices." It's usually not that terrible. The American ideal of self-reliance, praised by Ralph Waldo Emerson, should not be confused with the willful ignoring of danger signals, burying your head in the sand like an ostrich. It is part of human nature to deny the possibility of bad things happening, but denial is as bad as excessive worry. Everyone needs some introspection in identifying what the real worries are, and what one's weaknesses are.

Your health care can be seriously compromised by a tactical error. It is a good idea to think about what approach you take in seeking your own care, based on your knowledge of human nature. If you adamantly demand service (not merely request it), you may be more likely to get it, while perhaps meeting resistance, but you will surely get less cooperation on your next visit.

Weigh Your Options

You may not have much choice of health-care plans, but when you do, gather as many facts and ideas as possible, and weigh your personal preferences and needs. No matter how carefully thought out your decision may be, time and circumstances may change, and in any case everyone should have a fallback plan or alternative.

If you have choices, and after carefully looking at your own assets and liabilities, it may seem best to buy merely catastrophic insurance, that is, a health-insurance policy with a high deductible of $2,000, $3,000, or more, assuming that one can take care of the smaller expenses. No one but the very richest people can pay for catastrophic illness. Others, with iron self-discipline, might be able to set aside in savings a very large "sickness" fund. Even an older person if he or she has conscientiously saved the money that would have gone into paying for a health plan, may still come out ahead. Finally, many people, whether through choice or circumstances, have no health insurance and have no plan to achieve it. This "going bare" may seem to be satisfactory to some young people for a long period of time. They are willing to take chances on never becoming ill or injured, unrealistic though this may be, trusting that under disastrous circumstances someone else may pick up the bills. I do not advise this solution. There are, at present, over 40 million Americans with no health insurance at all according to Paul Starr of Princeton University, one of the most widely read and quoted students of health care. It seems to me that this is a recipe for disaster not only for these people, but for the nation.

When trying to assess a new doctor or health plan, or alternative treatment, sometimes there is no substitute for actually making an appointment and making a visit. Beware of the medical practice or group that puts pressure on you, the prospective patient, to sign up at the first visit for a long course of treatment, be it exercise, chiropractic, or transcendental meditation. People who have nothing to hide will disclose the information that you need and will not insist on your signing up in advance for an expensive course of treatment.

On January 14, 1996 the *New York Times* had these suggestions for picking an HMO:

1. What percentage of the plan's network doctors are board certified, and what percentage leave the plan each year?
2. If the plan has a "quality report card" or has been audited by the National Committee for Quality Assurance or other organization, inspect the report.
3. What's in the sample benefits contract?

4. How many complaints filed with the state insurance department against the plan have been upheld?
5. Must primary care physicians receive permission from the HMO before making referrals to specialists? And for women, does that rule include gynecologists?
6. How easy is it to file an appeal when medical treatment is denied?
7. What portion of the plan's premium dollars is spent on medical care?
8. If possible, find out what sort of financial incentives doctors receive for holding down the cost of medical care.
9. What type of preventive care, such as immunizations, does the plan offer?
10. What kind of preauthorization is needed for hospitalization?
11. Is a prescription drug you regularly take on the plan's list of medications approved for payment?

Newsweek magazine on June 24, 1996, published two cover stories: "America's Best HMOs," with their ratings of 43 plans, and "How to Choose Your Doctors," emphasizing some of the same points made in this book. *Newsweek*'s estimate of the number of Americans now in HMOs is 103.2 million, and describes this system as the "Wal Mart model of health care."

Likewise, when choosing a doctor, after weighing the various aspects mentioned in chapter 3, the decision will usually be the result of a combination of availability, reputation, affordability, and your own personal preference. The primary-care physician you choose for yourself may not take care of children, so if you have children, you will have to go through the same processes to select a pediatrician. Finding a doctor for your adolescent children is always ticklish. Adolescents usually resent having to continue on with their "baby doctor," but often there is a bond with a pediatrician that lasts for a lifetime. Many adolescents, even young adults, continue to go back to their pediatrician by choice. Whether or not this pediatrician feels competent and willing to go on with treating your adolescent child needs to be discussed. Most pediatricians are trained in adult medicine as well. The training of medical students today, and the further training in pediatrics and family practice residency programs, incorporates knowledge of the problems of adolescence as a separate topic worthy of close attention.

The physician who has been selected by the patient or by the plan may not turn out to be the best choice. So much depends on the ability of the patient to communicate with the doctor; sometimes great personality differences result in frustration for both parties. If the situation is thoroughly unsatisfactory, then the patient should change his or her doctor, and all health plans should make this possible, although many do not. Find this out before you sign up with any plan. Likewise, if you are in a managed-care plan and have not been able to achieve a satisfactory resolution of such things as chronic lower back pain, or chronic headache, then it is not a bad idea to consider some of the alternative approaches to health care, to explore what options are available, difficult as they may be to evaluate.

There are some circumstances under which free care may be available. Hospitals that have received federal funding—and almost all of them have—are obligated by law to give a certain amount of free care. Your local Senior Action Council, Welfare office, Social Security office, or chapter of AARP can supply details. Obviously, to make such an arrangement work the hospitals or emergency rooms must have definite evidence of the patient's inability to pay. In addition, the agency called Emergency Aid to Elderly, Disabled, and Children (EADC), provides for free care in emergencies for these people (again if the patient can demonstrate an inability to pay). This program is administered separately in each state, and your local Social Security office can provide appropriate information. The paperwork involved in applying for such assistance is lengthy and complicated. Many patients give up in the face of a pile of hard-to-understand forms, and all physicians find that filling out their portion of these forms is time-consuming, and often that the information requested is not available.

Veterans are entitled to free care for service-connected disabilities. The custom of giving free care to the clergy went out of style many years ago, although many individual physicians still offer it. "Professional courtesy" whereby physicians treated other doctors without charge has also largely disappeared due to specialization and to the fact that most physicians now have health-care coverage for themselves.

Many large pharmaceutical firms have plans to give medication at sharply reduced prices or free under certain conditions. This requires a note from a doctor with the diagnosis, and a statement that the patient is in financial need. Under some circumstances patients on Medicaid can receive prescriptions free. The fifty drug manufacturers who participate in the indigent prescription program have a income ceiling of $25,000 per individual, $40,000 for a couple, and the program covers some 270 drugs. Each state department of welfare or Department of Public Health has information on the details. Patients seeking these savings often meet with some bureaucratic resistance and need to do a lot of legwork.

Another choice facing everyone is whether to insist on the brand-name medication or to accept a generic substitute. The Food and Drug Administration carries out a rather complete surveillance of brand-name drugs, but such surveillance is not possible for all generics, which are too often made outside of the United States by small, relatively unknown companies. The passage of generic-drug legislation in many states several years ago was based on a good intention, which was to provide the cheapest possible reliable medicine for a given illness. In Massachusetts, for example, pharmacists are required to supply the generic unless the physician specifically writes "no substitution" on the prescription form. Human nature being what it is, ways have been found to make this situation profitable. A pharmacy or a chain can buy generic drugs at the lowest possible price, but it is not required to sell them for the lowest possible price. Thus they may actually achieve a much larger profit margin by supplying a generic. Most managed-care plans now have a formulary that gives the relative costs of various brand names of each drug and their equivalents in generics. Pressure is put on the physicians to prescribe the least expensive drug of comparable quality. Some third-party insurers have arranged with certain pharmacy chains to supply prescription drugs at a discount, sometimes by requiring a co-payment. This has been a welcome step forward in controlling the costs.

Another decision to be made is whether to use a community hospital or a teaching hospital. Having considered the nature of both, the choice must be made after weighing all the many factors discussed in chapters 3, 4, and 6. There are relatively few conditions that can be taken care of only in large metropolitan teaching hospitals. Every year some magazines rate the "best hospitals in America" usually based on subjective judgments by physicians surveyed. These guidelines are fairly reliable if you are seeking the best in specialized, highly technological care. In human terms, the ratings may be quite different. Common sense should tell you that to have, for example, a simple hernia repair performed by a competent local doctor in the small hospital in your community should be a satisfactory experience. Common sense should also tell you that you would not expect to have open-heart surgery done in such a small facility. Managed-care plans like to have the patients go to the community hospitals because the daily cost is lower. To stay in existence, university hospitals often contract with managed-care plans to take care of the plan's patients at a lower fixed rate, but this practice increases the likelihood that they will accumulate operating deficits and face impending closure. In the best managed-care plans with which we are familiar, the quality of care may not be sacrificed to save money, but the pressure on doctors and caregivers to do so is always present.

You'll be able to make better decisions about health care if you inform yourself about health developments and issues. There are almost numberless excellent resources available to those interested in their health. Magazines for women and magazines for health-and-fitness enthusiasts are full of advice that is for the most part useful and reliable. There are several very good books on general health and disease available to the general public, a few of which are listed under References. Health letters are published at regular intervals by institutions such as Harvard Medical School, Stanford Medical School, the Mayo Clinic, and Johns Hopkins School of Medicine. Most public libraries have several of these useful references.

Develop a Health-Care Strategy

The term "strategy" was primarily used in the past to describe a battle plan as part of a campaign. This may be an appropriate model for achieving good health care. Having read about the setting, the players, the operating system, and some of the pitfalls, the reader has by now made an assessment of these factors and we hope has reflected on the process of making decisions.

GET ORGANIZED

Keep a complete and up-to-date file of your and your family's health information. This should include complete information on the health of every member of the family, including immunizations, with reference to the date it was administered, where, and by whom. Physicians are now required to record the manufacture and lot number of immunizations and to provide patients with an information sheet on the good and bad effects of the vaccine. Families should keep a record of all major illnesses and operations. The names and addresses of physicians and hospitals where major events took place are easily forgotten. Records of allergies to natural substances and to medicines are vitally important. Dangerous and sometimes even fatal reactions to various drugs have occurred when known allergies were not recorded and the information not passed on.

Old medical reports from previous doctors or hospitalizations are invaluable. It is well to record the date of surgical operations, the final diagnosis, and the name of the surgeon. All too often physicians have difficulty finding out about these past events, which may be critically important in diagnosing the present illness. The patient often seems to suppress the memory of an unpleasant illness, and to ignore its implications. When transferring the medical care of any member of the family to a new doctor or group, it is important not only to have the old records sent to the new doctor, but equally important to keep a copy of the records at home.

Many private and group practices and all managed-care plans have printed information with regulations, hours, charges, and mechanisms for making appointments. Keeping this written information on file at home will save you time and trouble. People who make an appointment and don't keep it add to the cost of delivery care. In managed-care plans this "no show" rate varies from 1 percent to 20 percent. Various mechanisms exist to discourage this behavior or even penalize patients. This should be spelled out in plan literature. If the printed material does not contain information on the mechanisms for requesting referral to a specialist or a request for a second opinion, then it is a good idea to secure this information before illness strikes. The same may be said for a written statement on the procedures for appealing denial of a specialist referral or second opinion. It goes without saying that the telephone numbers of the doctors, the hospital, the health-plan manager, and the emergency room need to be kept not only in the file, but probably posted by the home telephone.

The next aspect of the strategic plan has to do with money. It may be hard to get a straightforward, simple written list of costs and charges for medical care from the doctor or group enrolled in an indemnity plan or from the managed-care plan (HMO or other). The money contributed by the patients may be only part of the total payment, the rest coming from an employer or from Medicare or other government agencies. Some of these costs may be recouped on the income-tax return and others not. A record of expenses should include all out-of-pocket expenses for health care, particularly for alternative treatments outside of the prepaid system, and all medications. This is useful for reviewing in considering your health plan and even more useful in recording deductions that may be taken on an income-tax return. Having made the choice of plan, it is important to remember that not everything will be covered and some expenses will have to be paid out of pocket, so accumulating some savings is or should be part of your health-care planning. This is particularly true if you intend to look into forms of alternative care. In some of the plans currently proposed in Congress, each tax-payer would be allowed a credit or actual payment voucher that would go toward buying either one of the standard medical-care plans or alternative medical care. These proposed "medical savings accounts" would be interest-bearing and tax-free.

TAKE CARE OF YOURSELF

After we have spent much time in worrying about illness, suffering, and death we need to hear some comforting words. There is more reason for optimism than pessimism. Everyone needs to be reminded that most infectious diseases are self-limited. Sprains, superficial scratches, and bruises also heal themselves. Simple remedies are the best for tension headaches, diarrhea, and epidemic gastroenteritis.

Regular physical examinations are reassuring to many people, although statistically it is difficult to prove that the annual well-person checkup of the adult without symptoms yields a significant savings in health-care costs.

To ensure better health, you'll want to begin a regular regime of moderate exercise. As far as cost-effectiveness in preventive health care is concerned, vigorous walking is both cheap and effective in terms of cardiovascular health. The best motivation for regular exercise is enjoyment. To work out doggedly because it is the thing to do usually leads a person to taper off or even to abandon the program. Golfing can be a wonderfully enjoyable excuse for walking, but the crowding of popular courses has led to the widespread use of golf carts, a sedentary practice that speeds up the game. Health clubs have facilities to accomodate any range from mild to heavy exercise. It is wise to use their advice on the level of exertion you should attempt, after preliminary training. Some clubs require a doctor's certificate of fitness; others make their own evaluation. Home exercise machines, ranging in price from $100 to $1000, can help you try to achieve and maintain good cardiovascular fitness and a sense of well-being. Swimming is an excellent exercise, particularly suitable for people with hip, back, or knee disease which might be made worse by walking or cycling. But there are some people who either cannot or will not exercise. If they are not obese, and have good genes, they may live as long as the exercisers. Jogging, even distance running, after medical clearance and using proper equipment (not necessarily the most expensive) brings pleasure and a high degree of fitness to millions of Americans, but many people get the most exercise and the most satisfaction at home, in gardening, doing household repairs, even moving furniture and house painting. The essence is that any form of exertion should be done with gusto, leading to some sense of satisfaction.

Nutrition is so widely discussed, in magazines, in lectures, on the radio and television, that nobody can plead ignorance. Currently the consensus of experts is that the diet should be low in fat, containing five fruits or vegetables daily and an adequate amount of protein. There is less agreement about the proper amounts of meat, salt, milk, and eggs in the diet. The new labeling of food products instituted by the FDA helps all of us make more informed decisions about what to eat. With a proper diet and normal digestion there is no proven need for added vitamins. The experts tell us that fast foods and snacks tend to be high in fats, sugars, artificial colors, and artificial flavors, but they are easily and quickly obtainable, and most people think they taste good, so they buy these foods in huge quantities. It should be a matter of serious concern to all of us that many Americans—perhaps as many as a quarter of us—cannot afford the recommended fruits, vegetables, meat, and milk for themselves or for their children.

Proper nutrition is not inconsistent with the moderate use of alcohol, and some studies seem to show that there are definite beneficial effects to the circulation from drinking moderate amounts. What is moderate? Probably four ounces of wine, six or eight ounces of beer, or two ounces of hard liquor would meet most definitions of moderate. Of course, some conditions, notably alcoholism, positively contraindicate any use of alcohol whatsoever.

And as far as I am concerned, as an ex-smoker, nothing good can be said about smoking. Smoking is a powerful addiction, very difficult to overcome, as I know from personal experience and the experiences of many patients. Sad to say, most smokers know that they are doing themselves serious, possibly fatal harm by continuing with the habit. It is fashionable at present to blame the giant tobacco companies for pushing their product and for blocking legislative curbs on tobacco sales, but human nature is partially to blame as well. Teenagers face peer pressure to take up smoking. Many who resent being told how to behave by parents, teachers, or legislators smoke in defiance to prove their independence. Many male laborers feel that smoking is a manly way of asserting their scorn for academics and the wealthy, who by and large are increasingly nonsmokers. Many more young women smoke at present, perhaps more so than young men of their own social groups, possibly as a way of asserting their equal rights. The psychology that leads people to smoke and the power of nicotine addiction do not give us cause for optimism that tobacco smoking will disappear in this country.

You'll also need to be prepared to seek out the support you need to handle illnesses, injuries, or other conditions that affect your health. Almost any ailment or health-related problem is more easily borne if you have support from people who care, who understand that particular problem, and who will listen. Some people find support by joining health clubs. There are now innumerable support groups for various illnesses and health conditions, usually led by nonprofessionals but often with trained special input. Traditionally such support has come from clergy, or church-sponsored groups, but now lay leadership is by far the commonest. Others gain support by joining Alcoholics Anonymous, Al-Anon, Narcanon, and other similar organizations. To take an outstanding example, Alcoholic Anonymous (AA), an American innovation less than sixty years old, has developed principles that help guide people in improving their life situations. Probably more alcoholics have been helped to sobriety through AA than through all medical and psychiatric methods combined. The anonymity is partly a device to protect the alcoholic from social or occupational threats. Meeting daily, weekly, or monthly with a number of like-minded people using confession, education, and encouragement produces good, but not perfect, results. The principle of helping others is at the heart of this and other self-help organizations.

Weight Watchers and Smoke Enders give support to those enmeshed in the never-ending struggles against obesity and nicotine. For people over fifty-five, membership in the American Association of Retired Persons (AARP) not only brings a magazine, *Modern Ma-*

turity, with frequent excellent articles on the preservation of health, but maintains a pharmacy ordering service that can bring members savings in prescribed drugs. Most local television stations and national networks have health advisors who regularly come on the air to express opinions, which usually are a reflection of current research findings and teachings.

In your planning it helps to think hard about, and then to list, those conditions for which you really do not need to go to the clinic or the doctor. These include waiting a reasonable period of time to see if some bothersome but not disabling, self-limiting conditions heal of themselves. These might include head colds, gastroenteritis, temporary insomnia, bruises, sprains, headaches, and toothaches. It takes judgment and a certain amount of luck to decide how long you can take care of yourself without help, but that certainly is what must occur if we wish to reserve our costly medical facilities for those with demonstrated need. Self-reliance, based on knowledge, seems to be the wave of the future.

11

The Future of Health Care

*We should all be concerned about the future because
we will have to spend the rest of our lives there.*

CHARLES F. KETTERING

Historically, medical education has been slow to change with the
times. Patients, as well as doctors, will have to change their expectations and become better informed about the maintenance of health
for themselves and their families. In the future we face exceedingly
complex issues that will shape medical care. Dr. M. R. Greenlick, in
the March 1995 issue of the journal *Academic Medicine,* provides a
useful summary and reasonable prediction of the changes in the
structure of the health-care system (see table, next page).

The changes since 1935 are profound, but dramatic shifts have
taken place in the past ten years. Both physicians and laymen may
be out of touch, and, indeed, out of sympathy, but there can be no
going back to the good old days, which were really not that good.
The changes in the way in which doctors practice and the way they
are paid are well known. The replacement of the hospital as the

Changes in the Structure of the Health Care System in One Lifetime

	1935	1985	2005
Nature of practice	Solo practice	Small to med.-sized organized forms	Large organizations
Payment mechanism	Out of pocket	Private insurance and out of pocket	Socially organized payment mechanisms
Dominant site of care	Doctor's office	Hospital	Diffuse networks
Role of government	None	Payer of last resort	Primary organizer of financing
Form of physician payment	Fee for service	Mixed	Capitation and salary
Role of technology	Minimal	Moderate—mostly hospital	Extremely high
Function of medical care	Care	Curing disease	Disease prevention—maintenance of function
Measured by	How nice?	How technical?	How cost-effective?
Physician obligation to patients	1:1	Ambiguous	$1:n$

dominant site of care has been explained in chapters 4 and 6. The move toward ever-greater technological changes cannot and should not be reversed. Prevention of illness and maintenance of fitness have been preached by professional authorities for years, but it has taken the dollars-and-cents demonstration of the cost savings of prevention and early intervention to bring about a widespread acceptance. The last two lines of Dr. Greenlick's table are the most disturbing to most of us. In the future the relief of pain and suffering will often be measured in terms of cost-effectiveness. Assigning dollar values to care is, and will be, nearly impossible. As regards the feelings of physicians toward treating their patients as an obligation, a duty, and a privilege, professionals and the public will have to be educated and mutually tolerant and trusting. This is a very large prescription.

As the number of older people continues to increase, many thoughtful students of health care have suggested cutting down on the costly medical care of later life. Actual rationing so far has principally taken the form of limiting the upper age for such heroic measures as organ transplantation and open-heart surgery, both formally and by unwritten consensus. Actually, several recent studies have cast doubt on the magnitude of health-care costs for the aged. There are some who believe old people have "a duty to die," but many of these believers change their minds as they themselves age. In my experience, many old people do indeed feel they have lived a full life and are ready to go, but they cannot help living on. Honest discussion of these issues becomes highly emotional. The cost to taxpayers is always a consideration, but it is not often openly admitted or faced realistically, particularly in an election year. In all likelihood someday a uniform policy of health care for the aged will be developed, but the discussion of how to finance it will be long and heated. We have seen that Americans over the age of sixty-five receive much more costly medical care than in other countries. The desire of the managed-care plans and the public to save money will be stronger than the profit motivation of manufacturers and the personal preferences of practitioners. The costs of terminal care and of the elderly will undoubtedly be restricted to some degree and in some form. Whether or not these entitlements are to be cut back will be the next great battle in the health-care debate. Realistically, this problem will not be resolved in the near future. At present it is almost certain that there will be fewer subsidized services available to older people. For that reason people should make their own old-age plans, going on the assumption that the government will not take care of them.

The capitalistic system depends on generating "need." Medical discoveries, publicity, as well as health-care articles and television shows, have generated increased utilization and demand. So increased demand is going to be another battleground. The managed-care plans will continue to try to decrease the provision of costly services so as to ensure continued profits, but the profits of the pharmaceutical industry will continue to stimulate advertising and publicity, which in turn will stimulate demand for more and newer drugs, and more highly technological treatments.

Money and costs will continue to be all important in the eventual health-care decisions the government makes, as well as the health plans employers, individuals, and their families select. If there is government-mandated universal coverage, which certainly seems an essential goal, it will probably make provisions for payment, or at least co-payment, for those many Americans who choose alternative treatment outside of the established system. Alternative therapies will probably be regulated by the newly established branch of the National Institutes of Health, which is at present studying and evaluating various alternative systems of treatment.

Practice will be different for your doctors and nurses and other health-care workers. More practice guidelines will be developed that will not be mandatory but will aim at better quality and more cost-effective health care. Failure to practice within published guidelines will become less acceptable, affording protection to patients but imposing some lack of flexibility on their care. The prescribing physician will have fewer options and may be penalized for prescribing patterns not listed in a plan's formulary, which is a list of the least-expensive effective drugs. Generalists will be rated according to the number of tests they order and the number of specialty referrals they make. Primary-care doctors will have more training in the specialties. Reports of reprimands or other disciplinary actions for doctors and nurses will become more and more a matter of public record. Physicians in general will have lower incomes, but excellent benefits for health insurance, continuing medical education, and malpractice coverage. There will be strong financial incentives for health-care workers to move to underserved areas such as the inner cities and remote rural areas. This will come about by such incentives as government financing of medical-student education, and provision for these doctors of first-rate health-care facilities. There will be efforts to pay for the medical education of doctors, and residency training, out of tax funds, in return for prescribed periods of various types of public service. This system has worked well in other countries and in our own National Health Service Corps. Physicians and nurses will have to master information retrieval in the face of ever-expanding scientific knowledge, because it is impossible for them to keep in their heads all of the details of new medications, new diagnostic tools, and new legal requirements.

The managed-care organizations will continue to improve on their recruiting of primary-care physicians. We hope they will make available to prospective patients as much information as possible about their doctors. With luck, patients and physicians who are a good match will find each other. Word of mouth recommendations from friends and other physicians will always be the best way of finding the right doctor within the system. Trained and sympathetic nurse practitioners have already been embraced by patients who have accepted their competence in dealing with medical problems. Nurse practitioners will do more and more of the primary care.

Already, managed-care plans, as noted, place heavy responsibilities on primary-care physicians for sorting, rerouting, and managing complex matters themselves in person or by telephone. These duties are going to continue to place increasing strain on primary-care physicians, and the liability incurred by these heavy responsibilities will increase. We will not see any increased number of physicians going into primary care unless their workload is evened out and their financial compensation matches that of the specialists. The number of physicians in this country is now about 700,000. Estimates of the number of physicians we would need if all Americans joined HMOs are usually about 500,000 or fewer, because of the greater productivity (that is, the large patient load) for the primary-care doctors, and the reduction in specialist referrals.

What does the future hold for you, the patient? There will be more AIDS, more drug-resistant bacterial infections, new viruses, epidemics of influenza with new strains of viruses, more old people, probably more violence and acts of civil disorder, and probably more substance abuse. There will continue to be unexpected natural disasters: earthquakes, fires, famine, floods, hurricanes, and droughts. On the brighter side, there will be more complete childhood immunizations, fewer cesarean sections, fewer referrals to specialists, and less "defensive" laboratory testing. The decreased number of hospitalizations and shorter stays in the hospital are already here and will continue to be emphasized. There will be fewer hysterectomies, circumcisions, and breast implants.

There will be more, rather than less, governmental involvement in health care. There must be, because, as we have seen, the health of the public involves supporting, enforcing, and administering immunizations for all, and securing safe drinking water, air, and food supplies. These functions have traditionally been in the providence of federal, state, and local boards and commissions. These responsibilities cannot and should not be delegated to the profit-oriented private sector. The current vogue of government bashing has already begun to erode some of our essential safeguards by reducing the allotments for basic health-protection services. The government—local, state, and federal—is essential for maintaining those functions that defend against these threats to our health, including extreme poverty, epidemics, malnutrition, poor housing, and joblessness. This is not just "do-good liberalism." It is a realistic and hard-headed approach to the stability of this country. Instead of bashing government and scorning politics and politicians, we can hope that more citizens will work at the local level involving themselves in these issues. Inept politicians only flourish when the average citizen is apathetic, blind to the future of his children.

Your doctor will be well trained, and the practice of general and specialty medicine will be more closely supervised and uniform. For that reason the choice of physician (if you have any choice) will be based on your personal preferences, as the quality of care will be more reliable because managed-care programs can select and oversee well-trained doctors. The oversupply of physicians at present will inevitably lead to greater competition for positions in the health-care organizations. In the near future any would-be patient will be able through computer data to know more about the various plans available. In Minnesota, a consortium of managed-care plans has established a data bank, whereby a potential consumer can find the location of various plans, their characteristics, the names of their doctors, their specialties, and their performance profiles. Such databases will probably become a national trend.

The future of hospitalization for mental illness is clearly visible in what has already happened under managed care. Formerly, patients stayed for months, even years, and the pace of therapy was relatively leisurely. Many people paid the tremendous costs out of pocket. Others up to now have been covered by some of the better indemnity plans, such as Blue Cross/Blue Shield, but these generally had a limit of from thirty to ninety days of hospitalization. The federal government employees' health insurance has for many years provided almost unlimited payment to federal employees for mental health, but those benefits also have been sharply curtailed and will be even more sharply curtailed in the future. The exodus of psychiatrists from private practice is already well underway, and there will be few, indeed, who can be supported by direct, nonreimbursed payments by private patients. The handling of patients in mental hospitals will continue to resemble more and more that of the general hospitals. That is, patients will not be admitted except on demonstration of severe need. The period of evaluation is already much shorter than in the past, and will be even shorter. Patients, in most cases, will be staying probably only a matter of days or a very few weeks for the sickest. The average stay at the McLean Hospital near Boston, one of the country's most renowned private mental institutions, now averages fourteen days, as opposed to many months in the past. State mental institutions will then take on the unreimbursed burden of those who are seriously mentally ill and simply unable to exist outside of an institution.

The criterion for admission will be "medical necessity," and the decision on the validity of such a claim will be made by someone working for the managed-care plan who has not seen the patient and who may not even be medically trained. Dr. Leonard Glass, a psychiatrist, has referred to managed care as the "health-care-denial industry." More seriously disturbed people will of necessity be looked after by their families. Inevitably there will be disastrous outcomes, such as suicide or violent assaultive behavior. The backlash to this will undoubtedly put great pressure on health-care plans to be more liberal about mental hospitalization. Until such a reversal takes place, the families of the mentally ill may expect their loved ones to be treated at these "McDonald's of Mental Health," as they have been called.

The criteria of cost-effectiveness will be applied to psychotherapy of all sorts, and to physical therapy, nutrition, podiatry, and the routine checkup of healthy children and adults. The routine well child or adult checkup will rely more and more on data gathered by assistants and placed in the computer (perhaps even entered by the patients themselves). Your records will be computerized and much more complete than in the past. This information will be available to your doctor, which is a good thing, but there will undoubtedly be some loss of confidentiality, as many people will have access to a mass of computerized data. There will be battles to establish the true cost-effectiveness of some treatments such as those dealing with mental-health problems, behavior disorders, and substance abuse, which impose huge hidden costs on society. As the cost cutters curtail the number and types of services offered, expenditures will increase in hospitals, sanitariums, and correctional institutions. State and federal agencies will be forced to pick up these costs through tax revenues.

As more care will be carried out by generalists, and referral to specialists will thereby be restricted, the increased responsibility will bring more incentive for malpractice suits. Malpractice awards will probably be limited in size; legislation for that purpose is now before state and federal legislatures. At present American physicians work an average of fifty-seven hours a week, according to extensive surveys and self-reported studies carried out by the American Medical Association. If physicians under managed care follow a more corporate lifestyle approaching a forty-hour workweek, then clearly we will need many more medical-school graduates, unless those now entering specialties become generalists in the employ of managed-care plans.

There will be several kinds of disincentives for inappropriate use of the emergency room—probably a system of financial penalties. The patient will be informed that his or her recent visit to an emergency room was not authorized in advance, and that the plan's review concluded that the visit was not a true emergency. In that case, the patient will then be responsible for the emergency-room bill. For this policy to work will require, of course, better arrangements for prompt care of nonurgent complaints.

There will, I hope, be expansion of the system already in place in some hospitals whereby the emergency room is linked with a walk-in or urgent-care clinic, staffed around the clock. Ideally, the emergency room could refer the nonemergency patients to their own primary doctor or practice group and use this urgent-care center only for the uncovered. Each person, we may hope, will have a primary-care physician or nurse practitioner, ideally working together. By making primary-care service available around the clock, the emergency room will be reserved for true emergencies.

Managed-care plans will continue to develop formularies requiring the use of the least-expensive drugs available for various conditions. The desire of the managed-care plans and the public to save money will be stronger than the profit motivation of manufacturers and the personal preferences of practitioners. The pharmaceutical manufacturers will claim that people are thus denied freedom of choice. Some practitioners will continue to have strong feelings of brand loyalty; many cardiologists, for example, insist on the brand name Lanoxin in place of the generic digoxin.

It will still be possible, although increasingly expensive, to buy independent indemnity health insurance in order to continue the custom of going to the physician of one's choice, and paying for each service at the time, with some degree of insurance coverage. In general though, the option of choosing one's own fee-for-service doctor will virtually disappear, especially in urban areas. At present, indemnity payments or fee-for-service medicine are still available to Medicare patients and their physicians. With all of the present concern about the runaway costs of Medicare, however, it is almost certain that all Medicare patients will be put into one or another sort of managed-care plan, and will not have the freedom of choice of physicians and hospitals that they now possess. Already, people on Medicaid in many places have been arbitrarily assigned to closed-panel, managed-care plans.

Currently payment will not be made for, nor will managed-care systems provide, untried or alternative therapies, although future health-care legislation might take this into consideration. Each therapy will have to demonstrate its cost-effectiveness to be accepted. It is possible that those who wish to stay out of the regular health-care system can have instead a system of payment that could be applied to alternatives.

As more people are turned off by their ten-minute physical examination and the denials of specialist consultation, there will be legislative curbs and public demand for less emphasis on profit. The huge profits of managed-care systems, and the enormous salaries of their nonmedical C.E.O.'s will inevitably bring calls for reasonableness and fairness. Consumer groups will form and demand power in shaping health-care delivery. Politicians, always with an eye on the polls, will slowly act on these demands despite intense lobbying by those profiting from the present system.

More and more, patients will have access to medical information that they did not have before, as a result of on-line communications such as the Internet and America Online. Up to now the structure of medicine has largely been based on the assumption that the physician has all of the information and the patient must defer to the expert. Now the consumer can obtain virtually all information that the professionals have. This does not, of course, imply that the patient will be able to make a correct diagnosis of his or her own problems, nor select the best treatment, but the information certainly can be used as a guide to check on the reports and recommendations of the clinic, the specialist, or the primary-care doctor. Patient-doctor conversations that already in some cases resemble a dialogue or even a debate, rather than a one-sided authoritative plan, will continue to be a matter for individual negotiation. The patient will take a greater role in decision making. One implication of this is that the patient must at the same time accept some responsibility for the consequences. The physician in this circumstance will become more of a referral source, a persuader, and a negotiator.

The clinical faculty of medical-school teaching hospitals will be closely watched for productivity. Those who cannot bring in sufficient income generated by seeing many patients will be asked to leave. This cannot fail to have an impact on teaching and on clinical research, both of which are bound to suffer as the faculty practitioners will have to spend more time with patients. Tenure, which was originally instituted to offer job security to low-paid professionals, will be abolished. The power of hospital staffs has already been sharply reduced and will be reduced even further. The old power structure, says Dr. David Nash, is over. However, Dr. Carola Eisenberg of Harvard Medical School has pointed out that what we do as doctors is usually deeply gratifying regardless of the branch of medicine entered. She concluded by saying, "I cannot imagine a more satisfying calling. Let us make sure our students hear that message from us."

As to the future, we will clearly always need doctors and we will need hospitals for serious illnesses. We will continue to need highly specialized and technical procedures and the highly trained people to carry them out. Downsizing and consolidation of hospitals will undoubtedly continue at a frantic pace in order to save money.

There will come a time when services are reduced to an irreducible minimum, and downsizing will then cease. Psychoactive medicines will never completely replace the need for psychotherapy. Health-care costs will have been minimized, while many doctors, nurses, technicians, and aides will be out of work. The unanswered question is, whose money is saved? We will need to continue to take a hard look at the hidden costs of day surgery, of early hospital discharge after illness or delivery, and of reducing the ratio of nurses to patients. Here again active involvement by an informed public is needed.

Finally, do not despair. The numbers of outstanding young people who still want to be doctors and nurses continue to increase. People will still suffer, and will need help, but better delivery systems and better-trained, humane caregivers have the capability of bringing greater relief of suffering. Research will continue to bring about amazing revelations, new understanding, and new hopes. Putting all the pieces together will require time, thought, and a sense of fairness. One thing is certain: all aspects of health care will continue to be examined, debated, promoted, condemned, and altered. Those of the public who keep themselves informed and take more personal responsibility will do well, in sickness and in health.

Resource Guide

GENERAL MEDICAL INFORMATION

Agency for Health Care Policy and Research
Publications Clearinghouse
P. O. Box 8547
Silver Springs, MD 20907
(800) 358-4000

American Association of Osteopathic Specialists
804 Main Street, Suite D
Forest Park, GA 30050
(800) 447-9397

American Board of Medical Specialties
1007 Church Street, Suite 404
Evanston, IL 60201-5913
(800) 776-CERT

American Health Foundation
320 East 43rd Street
New York, NY 10017
(212) 953-1900

American Osteopathic Association
142 East Ontario Street
Chicago, IL 60610
(800) 621-1773

The American Self-Help Clearinghouse
St. Clares-Riverside Medical Center
25 Pocono Road
Denville, NJ 07834
(201) 625-7101

Center for Medical Consumers and Health Care Information
237 Thompson Street
New York, NY 10012
(212) 674-7105

Consumer Information Center
Pueblo, CO 81009
(719) 948-4000

Food and Drug Administration
Office of Consumer Affairs
5600 Fishers Lane, HFE-50
Rockville, MD 20857
(301) 443-3170

Health Care Financing Administration, Office of Public Affairs
U.S. Department of Health and Human Services
Hubert H. Humphrey Building, Room 435-H
200 Independence Avenue SW
Washington, DC 20001
(202) 690-6113
Medicare Hotline (800) 638-6833

233

Joint Commission on Accreditation of Healthcare Organizations
One Renaissance Boulevard
Oak Brook Terrace, IL 60181
(708) 916-5600

Medical Economics Magazine
Medical Economics Company
Montvale, New Jersey 07645
(201) 358-7200

National Health Information Center
P.O. Box 1133
Washington, DC 20013
(800) 336-4797

National Library of Medicine
National Institutes of Health
Bethesda, MD 20894
(800) 638-8480

National Organization for Rare Disorders
P.O. Box 8923
New Fairfield, CT 06812
(800) 999-NORD

National Self-Help Clearinghouse
Graduate School and University Center
   of the City University
   of New York
25 West 43rd Street, Room 6
New York, NY 10036

People's Medical Society
462 Walnut Street
Allentown, PA 18102
(215) 770-1670

Public Citizen Health Research Group
2000 P Street NW, 6th Floor
Washington, DC 20036
(202) 833-3000

SPECIFIC CONCERNS

Alzheimer's Disease Education and Referral Center (ADEAR)
P. O. Box 8250
Silver Springs, MD 20907

American Association of Retired Persons (AARP)
601 E Street NW
Washington, DC 20049
(800) 424-3410

American Coalition of Citizens with Disabilities
1012 Fourteenth Street NW, Suite 901
Washington, DC 20005
(202) 628-3470

American College of Nurse-Midwives
818 Connecticut Avenue NW, Suite 900
Washington, DC 20006
(202) 728-9860

Center for Environmental Health and Injury Control
Centers for Disease Control and
   Prevention (CDC)
Building 1, Room 2047
1600 Clifton Road NE
Atlanta, GA 30333
(404) 639-3286

Choice in Dying
200 Varick Street
New York, NY 10014
(800) 989-WILL

Clearinghouse on Family Violence Information
P.O. Box 1182
Washington, DC 20013
(703) 385-7565

Foundation for Hospice and Home Care
519 C Street NE
Stanton Park
Washington, DC 20002
(202) 547-6586

Hill-Burton Program
U.S. Department of Health and Human
    Services
5600 Fishers Lane, Room 11-25
Rockville, MD 20857
(800) 638-0742
(800) 492-0359

Midwives Alliance of North America
P.O. Box 175
Newton, KS 67114
(316) 283-4543

National Clearinghouse on Aging
Administration on Aging
330 Independence Avenue SW
Washington, DC 20201
(202) 619-0441

National Hospice Organization
1901 North Moore Street, Suite 901
Arlington, VA 22209
(800) 658-8898

National Lesbian and Gay Health Foundation
P.O. Box 65472
Washington, DC 20035
(202) 797-3708

ALTERNATIVE MEDICINE

American Botanical Council
P.O. Box 210660
Austin, TX 78720
(512) 331-8868

American Chiropractic Association
1701 Clarendon Boulevard
Arlington, VA 22209
(703) 276-8800

American Foundation for Alternative Healthcare, Research and Development
25 Landfield Avenue
Monticello, NY 12701
(914) 794-8181

American Foundation of Traditional Chinese Medicine
1280 Columbus Avenue, Suite 302
San Francisco, CA 94133
(415) 776-0502

American Holistic Medical Association
4101 Lake Boone Trail, Suite 201
Raleigh, NC 27607
(919) 787-5146

Association for Applied Psychophysiology and Biofeedback
10200 West 44th Avenue, Suite 304
Wheatbridge, CO 80033
(800) 477-8892

Committee for Freedom of Choice in Medicine
1180 Walnut Avenue
Chula Vista, CA 92011
(800) 227-4473

National Center for Homeopathy
801 Fairfax Street, Suite 306
Alexandria, VA 22314
(703) 548-7790

Office of Alternative Medicine
National Institutes of Health
6120 Executive Boulevard, EPS Suite
    450
Rockville, MD 20892
(301) 402-2466

OTHER RESOURCES

To find out what health-care providers
are in your local area, consult your
community's Chamber of Commerce
or your state's Better Business
Bureau. Also, contact Families
U.S.A. Foundation at 1334 G Street
NW, Washington, D.C. 20005.

To find out whether your plan is
accredited, contact the National
Committee for Quality Assurance at
(202) 955-3515.

Endnotes

INTRODUCTION

most important job. The nature of suffering and the goals of medicine, E. J. Cassell, New England Journal of Medicine, 306: 639–45, (March 18) 1982. The question of suffering and its relation to organic illness has rarely been addressed in the medical literature. This article offers a description of the nature and causes of suffering in patients undergoing medical treatment. A distinction based on clinical observations is made between suffering and physical distress.

CHAPTER 1

research. The Crisis in Clincal Research, E. H. Ahrens (New York: Oxford University Press, 1994). Discusses the shift away from the bedside.

basic health needs of its citizens. "Managed Care and the Morality of the Marketplace." J. P. Kassirer, *New England Journal of Medicine,* Editorial, 333:50, (July 6) 1995.

CHAPTER 2

decorum of the physical examination. "Can empathy be taught?" Howard Spiro, *Annals of Internal Medicine,* 116: 843, 1992.

when both parties proceed cautiously and politely. "How to talk to your doctor." Michelle Stacy, *Town and Country,* p. 78, July 1996. A straightforward approach, with practical suggestions.

Statistical Abstract of the United States. Issued annually by the Department of Commerce with countless statistics on a wide variety of topics. Because of the complexity of data gathering, the 1995 (latest) edition has figures from 1994 and even older.

CHAPTER 3

PSA controversy to the patient. "Screening for prostate cancer." W. A. Hensel, *New England Journal of Medicine,* 334: 667–8, (March 7) 1996. A practicing physician outlines the many time-consuming pieces of information expected, and in some cases legislated, of a doctor today.

cause of untold mischief." "Evaluation of Chest Pain in the Emergency Department." M. F. Stuman, *Annals of Internal Medicine,* 123: 317–8, (August 15) 1995. The author decries the pressures to do an excessive number of tests.

whether they are right." "Medicaid and managed care." J. K. Ingehart, *New England Journal of Medicine,* 332: 1727, 1995. The author quoted Dr. E. J. Cassell of Cornell Medical School and the Hastings Institute who has long been a student and advocate for assessing and teaching human values to the medical profession.

with more benefits and better salaries. A representative nursing service salary schedule has been in effect since 1992 at the Brigham and Women's Hospital in Boston. The minimum rate, for a beginning staff registered nurse is $18.37 per hour, and the maximum, for a clinical nurse specialist or midwife, after 15 years of continuous service, is $40.14 per hour. Rates vary throughout the United States, being somewhat higher in large cities, on both coasts.

has thrown nursing into a turmoil. "Money managers are unraveling the tapestry of nursing." E. D. Baer, *American Journal of Nursing,* 94:38–40, (October) 1994.

less qualified workers. "Map a new course for your career." Career Guide, *American Journal of Nursing,* (June) 1996, p. 8.

CHAPTER 4

and sore throat. "Medicaid Access Study Group: Access of Medicaid Recipients to Outpatient Care." A. L. Kellerman, *New England Journal of Medicine,* 330: 1426, 1994.

effects on people's health. "Rand Health Insurance Experiment. Health care for the poor. A public policy imperative." M. E. Whitcomb, *New England Journal of Medicine,* 315: 1220–2, (November 6) 1986. Large scale and thorough in scope. The basis for many subsequent plans.

1700 patients per doctor. "The Observer." *Newsletter of the American College of Physicians,* (March) 1995, p. 1.

with freedom of choice of doctor. "For Oxford Health, vital signs are fine." M. Brush, *New York Times,* Section 3, (March 31) 1996, p. 3.

welfare of patients. For a well-documented and rather angry detailed saga of one person's experiences with a well-regarded managed plan, read Casey Thomas's account entitled "HMO Overdose" in the April 10, 1995 issue of the *New Republic.*

let the patient beware." "Managing McLean." N. Miller, *Boston Globe Magazine,* September 10, 1995, p. 22.

Rhode Island alone. Human Service Yellow Pages. There is no national listing of such resources. As of 1996, The George D. Hall Company issued editions only for Massachusetts and Rhode Island.

rigidity and rules." "Managed Care: Ethical Issues." F. Rosner, *Journal of the American Medical Association,* Letter to the Editor, 274: 608–9, 1995.

CHAPTER 5

to provide them." Annual Report of the President, 1994. S. A. Schroeder, Robert Wood Johnson Foundation, Princeton, New Jersey.

his or her panel." "Physician compensation in the era of managed care." G. N. Herrle, *Medical Group Management Journal,* 39: 8–9, 1992.

July 1995. "Payment promises? Get them in writing." D. R. Sweeney, *Managed Care,* 4: 41–3, 1995.

colleagues in 1993. The Support of Medical Education. E. Ginzberg, The Josiah Macy Foundation, 1993.

according to the late Dr. Robert H. Ebert. In several personal conversations with the author, Dr. Robert H. Ebert described a study, necessarily anonymous, done at a prestigious eastern medical school within the last decade, over a four-year period. The figures were surprising to these researchers and publication of them without verification might have brought about a public outcry and a demand for lower public support for medical education by those unfamiliar with this complex field.

CHAPTER 8

not subject to government supervision or regulation. "Unconventional Medicine in the USA." D. M. Eisenberg, *New England Journal of Medicine,* 328: 246–252, 1993.

conventional or otherwise. "Bitter Herbs: Mainstream, Magic, and Menace." T. L. Delbanco, *Annals of Internal Medicine,* 121: 803–4, (November 15) 1994.

over 550 medicinal herbs . . . Herbs of Choice, *as reliable.* Madeline Drexler, *Boston Globe Magazine,* April 20, 1995.

CHAPTER 9

controversial and emotional. These progestational hormones or progestins are combined with estrogens in most oral contraceptives, as well as in hormone-replacement therapy.

surprisingly interesting reading. The Diagnostic and Statistical Manual of Mental Disorders. Abridged, 1994. A classification, with descriptions, that has been widely accepted both here and abroad and is useful in helping doctors and patients to be sure they are talking about the same thing.

CHAPTER 10

Wal Mart model of health care. "America's Best HMOs: How to Pick the Best Doctor." E. Spragins, *Newsweek,* June 24, 1996, 56–63.

quoted students of health care. The Social Transformation of American Medicine. P. Starr, New York, NY, Basic Books, 1984.

CHAPTER 11

and the patient does not. Drs. Thomas Ferguson and Warren Slack, Harvard Medical Center for Clinical Computing, 1995 and 1996. Personal communications.

our students hear that message from us. "It is Still a Privilege to be a Doctor." C. Eisenberg, *New England Journal of Medicine,* 314: 1113–4, (April 24) 1986.

The chart detailing changes in the health-care system is from an article by Dr. M. R. Greenlick, *Academic Medicine,* March 1995, Vol. 70: 179.

Bibliography

GENERAL INFORMATION

Consumer's Guide to Hospitals. Washington D.C.: Center for the Study of Services, 1995. Data on available services, size, costs, certification.

Miller, M. S. *Health Care Choices for Today's Consumers.* Washington D.C.: Living Planet Press, 1995. Up-to-date, objective, and reasonably complete.

Monagle, J. F., and D. C. Thomasma. *Health Care Ethics: Critical Issues.* Aspen, CO: Aspen Press, 1994.

"Sounding Board." *New England Journal of Medicine* 332 (1995): 465–68. A balanced look at health care reform from the point of view of the medical profession.

Starr, P. *The Social Transformation of American Medicine.* New York: Basic Books, 1984. The Classic Study, widely quoted.

Testa, M. A., and D. C. Simons. "Assessment of Quality of Life Outcomes." *New England Journal of Medicine* 334 (1996): 835–40. A detailed discussion of attempts to measure the quality of life in relation to health, a difficult but not impossible task. This may help you to formulate your own priorities.

United States Department of Commerce. *Statistical Abstract of the United States.* Washington D.C.: 1995. Annually updated data on innumerable topics.

THE ORGANIZATION OF MANAGED CARE

Bodenheim, T. S., and K. Grumbach. *Understanding Health Policy.* Stamford, CT: Appleton and Lange, 1995. Detailed, authoritative explanation, with case studies of various health care systems.

Brown, S. W., A. M. Nelson, S. J. Bronkesh, and S. D. Wood. *Patient Satisfaction Pays: Quality Service for Practice Success.* Frederick, MD: Aspen Press, 1993. Careful explanation of the cost-effectiveness of good quality medical care.

The Consumer's Guide to Health Plans. Washington D.C.: The Center for the Study of Services, 1994. Valuable data from an extensive survey of federal employees.

Gotcha, The Traps in Long Term Care Insurance. Yonkers, NY: Consumers Union of the United States, 1994. Look before you leap!

Hasan, M. H. "Let's End the Nonprofit Charade." *New England Journal of Medicine* 334 (1996): 1055–57. A doctor working for a for-profit, managed-care system attacks the performance of the nonprofits, not altogether convincingly.

Health Care Choices for Today's Consumer. Mt. Vernon, NY: Consumer Reports Books, 1995. Clear, uncomplicated outline of available choices.

Jacobsen, D., and E. D. Jacobsen. *Doctors are Gods.* New York: Thunder's Mouth Press, 1995. A critical look at doctors.

Nickerson, C. "Disgruntled Canadian Physicians Flock to U.S." *Boston Globe*, April 8, 1996. The dark side of the Canadian Health System, based on interviews with emigrating Canadian physicians.

Rosner, F. "Managed Care: Ethical Issues." Letter to the editor. *Journal of the American Medical Association* 274: (August 1995): 609–610.

Yarmolinsky, A. "Supporting the Patient." *New England Journal of Medicine* 332 (1995): 602–603. A professor of law and expert on medical economics has grave reservations about the motivation and ethical imperatives of investor-owned health care businesses.

SELF-HELP, SELF-CARE

American Medical Association Staff. *The American Medical Association Family Health Guide.* New York: Random House, 1987. Complete encyclopedic information for the public. An old standby.

Auerbach, P. S. *Medicine for the Outdoors.* Boston: Little, Brown, 1991. Useful for campers and those travelling on expeditions.

Berkeley Wellness Letter. University of California at Berkeley. Similar to the Harvard publication below. Several other medical schools have such letters.

Berkow, R., ed. *Merck Manual of Diagnosis and Theory.* Rahway, NJ: Merck Publishers, 1992. Time-honored encyclopedia of health and disease.

Candill, M. A. *Managing Pain Before It Manages You.* New York: Guilford, 1995. Useful and comprehensive discussion of pain management.

Complete Drug Reference: A Consumer Reports Book. Yonkers, NY: Published for the United States Pharmacopedia, 1996. Encyclopedic (750 pages) and authoritative. Details of every medication recognized by this organization.

Dixon, B. M. *Good Health for African Americans*. New York: Random House, 1994. Written from a particular perspective.

The Harvard Medical School Health Letter. Boston. Periodic reports on common problems, new research, medications, and advice.

Inlander, C. B. *The Consumer's Medical Desk Reference: Everything You Need to Know for the Best in Health Care*. Allentown, PA: Hyperion, 1995. Objective and thorough.

Krizmanic, J. *A Teen's Guide to Going Vegetarian*. New York: Puffin Books (Penguin), 1994. Useful if you have teenagers, or diet-conscious family members.

Mind-Body Institute. *The Wellness Book: The Comprehensive Guide to Maintaining Health and Treating Stress-Related Illness*. Boston: Deaconess Hospital, 1993. Relaxation, meditation, and other approaches.

Oppenheim, M. *A Doctor's Guide to the Best Medical Care*. New York: Wings Books, 1994. One of many such books, which are widely available.

Weil, A. *Spontaneous Healing*. New York: Knopf, 1995. Fair-minded, thorough, and containing some surprises.

WOMEN'S HEALTH

Carlson, K. J., Eisenstat, S. A., and Ziporyn, T., eds. *The Harvard Guide to Women's Health*. Cambridge, MA: Harvard University Press, 1996.

The Harvard Women's Health Watch. Boston. A monthly update on current issues.

Rosser, S. V. *Women's Health: Missing from U.S. Medicine*. Bloomington: Indiana University Press, 1994. Explanation of biases and omissions in health care.

Stewart, S. C., and Epps, R. P. *The Women's Complete Health Book*. New York: Delacorte Press, 1995. Multi-authored guide.

Women's Health Collective. *Our Bodies, Our Selves*. New York: Simon and Schuster, 1995. New edition of a pioneering and widely read book.

AGING, DEATH, AND DYING

Cohen, D., and C. Eisdorfer. *Caring for Your Aging Parents*. New York: Tucker/Putnam, 1995. Useful and comforting approach to a situation becoming more common all the time.

Kubler-Ross, Elizabeth. *On Death and Dying*. New York: Macmillan, 1993. The classic study.

Lieberson, A. J. *Advance Medical Directives*. New York: Clark, Boardman, Callaghan, 1995. Details and suggestions for preparing directives.

Migueis, J. R. *A Man Smiles at Death with Half a Face*. Hanover, NH: University Press of New England, 1990. A thoughtful, subjective account of a long illness and its effect on the patient and those around him.

ALTERNATIVE MEDICINE

"Chiropractors: Can They Help? Do They Harm?" *Consumer Reports*, June 1994. A thorough and objective review.

Eisenberg, D. M., et al. "Unconventional Medicine in the USA." *New England Journal of Medicine* 328 (1993): 246–52. Discussed in this book.

Lewith, G. T. "The Homeopathic Conundrum." *Journal of the Royal Society of Medicine* 83 (1990): 543–45. Summary of extensive studies in Great Britain.

Lockie, A., and N. Geddes. *The Complete Guide to Homeopathy*. New York: Dorling Kindersley, 1995. A sympathetic survey.

National Institutes of Health Report. *Alternative Medicine: Expanding Medical Horizons*. Washington D.C.: NIH of National Academy of Sciences, 1995. Outline of studies to be carried out. There are also many publications available on each alternative, strongly advocating it, and replete with anecdotal support.

"The Melatonin Craze," *Newsweek*, November 6, 1995. Even-handed summary.

Reid, Daniel. *A Handbook of Chinese Healing Herbs*. Boston: Shambhala Press, 1995. Extensive and enthusiastic.

SPECIFIC HEALTH-CARE CONCERNS:

Committee and Staff of the American College of Physicians. "Rural Primary Care: Position Paper of the American College of Physicians." *Annals of Internal Medicine,* 122 (March 1995): 381. Rural primary care contrasted with inner-city and suburban care.

Hilfiker, D. *Not All of Us Are Saints*. New York: Hill and Wang, 1994. Account of an articulate inner-city primary care physician.

Johnson, H. *Osler's Web*. New York: Crown, 1996. On the chronic fatigue syndrome. Critical of the medical establishment, but not up-to-date on current research.

Perts, T. T., and E. R. Wood. "Acute Care Costs of the Oldest Old." *Arch. Int. Med.* 15 (1996): 754–60. The authors say old people "cost less, their intensity is less, and they go to non-teaching hospitals." This contradicts the conventional wisdom.

Sin, A. I., et al. "Inappropriate Use of Hospitals in a Randomized Trial of Health Insurance Plans." *New England Journal of Medicine* 315 (1995): 1259–66. Cost-sharing (co-payments) did not reduce inappropriate hospitalization. In a study of 1,132 adults hospitalized in random trials, 23 percent of the admissions were "inappropriate" largely because of lack of a primary-care physician. Inability to meet co-payment earlier in an illness was also a factor.